Parenting Children with Diabetes

Parenting Children with Diabetes

A Guide to Understanding and Managing the Issues

ELIOT LEBOW

ROWMAN & LITTLEFIELD
Lanham • Boulder • New York • London

Published by Rowman & Littlefield
An imprint of The Rowman & Littlefield Publishing Group, Inc.
4501 Forbes Boulevard, Suite 200, Lanham, Maryland 20706
www.rowman.com

86-90 Paul Street, London EC2A 4NE

British Library Cataloguing in Publication Information Available

Library of Congress Cataloging-in-Publication Data

Names: LeBow, Eliot, 1971– author.
Title: Parenting children with diabetes : a guide to understanding and managing the issues / Eliot LeBow.
Description: Lanham : Rowman & Littlefield, [2019] | Includes bibliographical references and index.
Identifiers: LCCN 2019009913 (print) | LCCN 2019011163 (ebook)
Subjects: LCSH: Diabetes in children—Popular works. | Diabetes in children—Patients—Care. | Parents of chronically ill children. | Diabetic children.
Classification: LCC RJ420.D5 (ebook) | LCC RJ420.D5 L39 2019 (print) | DDC 618.92/462—dc23
LC record available at https://lccn.loc.gov/2019009913

ISBN: 978-1-5381-3120-6 (cloth : alk. paper)
ISBN: 978-1-5381-6389-4 (pbk. : alk. paper)
ISBN: 978-1-5381-3136-7 (electronic)

Contents

Introduction

Hi, my name is Eliot LeBow. I was diagnosed with type I diabetes in 1977 and then went on to become a diabetes-focused psychotherapist and certified diabetes educator. I would like to share with you and your family a part of my journey as well as what several of my clients have gone through while living with diabetes during childhood in order to educate others like you about what it feels like to have this disorder and what you may not understand as the parent of a child who has diabetes. I wrote this book for parents of children with diabetes and anyone who wants to gain insight into how it feels to have diabetes. I hope you learn a lot from my clients' experiences, feelings, and needs as children who grew up with this condition.

I designed this book as a guide to understanding what your family member or friend who lives with diabetes goes through on a daily basis and how you can help them. Through the recounting of various events in my clients' lives, I will share their feelings in the "Child's Perspective" sections. I will also give parental advice for how to maneuver through the challenges of raising a child with diabetes. For adults who grew up with or have diabetes, I provide insights into what you may have faced as a child—and what you still may be facing on a daily basis.

Growing up is difficult for everyone, but it is especially hard for children with diabetes in a world full of instant gratification. Chocolate, hard candy, soda, cotton candy, ice cream, cake, not to mention those Reese's peanut butter cups (mmmm). Oh, and let's not forget the ice cream man: Good Humor or Mister Softee, whichever one haunts your neighborhood, with his bell ringing and the truck that sings that unmistakable tune over and over again, beckoning every child on the block to come running out to meet him to buy and enjoy his or her treat. This is the nightmare of every child with diabetes—and it affects every parent of a kid living with diabetes. Relationships become strained and harder to keep intact for parents and their children due to fluctuating emotions, feelings of guilt, and other issues. Children with diabetes may feel different and isolated from their peers since they can't always eat the same things as everyone else at the same time. They may feel angry or sad, and even feel at times that it is their fault they got diabetes, as though getting it was punishment.

Oftentimes, the things we do as parents to protect our children from the dangers of the world become hurtful instead of helpful. This is especially true with children living with diabetes. Sometimes overprotecting or underprotecting while raising a child with diabetes can cause children to act out, leading to grave present and future consequences, including a wide range of physical issues and psychiatric disorders: attention deficit disorder (ADD), attention deficit/hyperactivity disorder (ADHD), learning disabilities, emotional problems, addictions, and others.

In the "Clinical Advice" and "Parental Advice" sections, I will help you to explore how improving the relationship between you and your child can successfully increase your child's ability to maintain good blood sugar control and reduce psychiatric, emotional, and educational problems. In some cases, this improvement may stop these problems from occurring altogether. Instead of protecting, maybe it would serve our children with diabetes better if we could be supportive of them during the issues they will have to face—some with you and others on their own.

The impact of poor diabetes management can take many forms, ranging from poor physical health to the loss of cognitive functioning.

It can also cause poor grades in school, which can lead to being placed in special education, causing more isolation and emotional upheaval. Children over time begin to feel helpless and that diabetes is not something that is manageable. Instead, it feels like more of a burden that prevents them from being normal. Other people in their surroundings may respond differently to them, like the school nurse, teachers, and camp counselors who feel they know what's right for the child with diabetes, even in many instances when they don't. Oftentimes, a child with diabetes will be told "you can't have any" when everyone else is being given candy or chocolate, needlessly isolating the child from their peers, when in fact a child with diabetes can eat sweets simply by adjusting his or her insulin. At home, a child may be punished by a parent for eating candy. This situation may cause the child to feel angry and frustrated—and the parent to feel guilty. As time goes by, the child may start isolating himself or herself from the family and his or her peers. Some other issues stemming from poor diabetes management include depression, low self-esteem, psychiatric disorders, low blood sugars, high blood sugars, and much more.

Since I was diagnosed with diabetes in 1977 at age six, I have had multiple learning disorders, experienced feelings of depression, and struggled with attention deficit disorder (ADD), all which I have managed to overcome in order to become an author, an abstract painter, and an expert in the field of psychotherapy for people with diabetes, as well as a well-rounded and overall happy person. In this book, I have chosen to share my clients' experiences, along with one or two of my own, with poor diabetes management and discuss how to help your child to avoid some of the pitfalls that have impacted their lives so he or she can grow up happy and healthy while learning to manage his or her diabetes.

1

The Day
Everything Changed

FRIDAY, JULY 16, 1982

It was a warm summer day, the kind with only a few puffy clouds in the crystal blue sky. John was six years old. His life was about to change forever, but to him it was exciting. Just ten days earlier, he had turned six years old. He lived in Gaithersburg, Maryland, on Tulip Grove Road in a nice, three-bedroom house with three stories, a deck, and a two-car garage on the corner of the block. You could enter through the kitchen or the living room. The bedrooms were on the top floor, and in the basement there was a recreation room and laundry room. His family's house was one of the first ones built in this community, which was surrounded by farms when they moved in four years earlier. Now that the community was complete, only three of the farms were left. In the back, there was a garden and a swing set with lots of land. John was a typical kid without a care in the world, and this house was his universe.

THE COOKIE MONSTER

He was so excited that his favorite babysitter was watching him today. She had promised to bring him a big plate of chocolate-chip cookies. He remembered watching her walk through the kitchen door and gently set a large plate covered in plastic wrap on the kitchen table. He ran up to the table and asked her if he could have some right there and then. She said, "John, you need to wait 'til lunch." His mom agreed.

Shortly after Mom left, John's babysitter opened the package on the table and called him into the kitchen. (*Note: This was the last time and last day that he would be allowed to have chocolate-chip cookies without a care in the world . . . without an argument, a negotiation, lying, or cheating. He didn't even know it yet. Wait! I'm getting a little ahead of myself.*) As John walked into the kitchen, she was standing there, holding a cookie in her hand as she said, "Happy birthday, dear! Enjoy as many as you want." He must have eaten at least ten large cookies in the first hour. He was so happy, and they were really good. His babysitter sat on the couch and watched TV most of the day as he played with his wooden blocks, Tonka trucks, and Tom, his cat. Tom was a fat, loveable, gray tabby who liked to lie in the sun in front of the living room window, and John loved lying there with him.

A few hours later, while lying with the cat, John noticed that he had to go to the bathroom to pee. Ten to fifteen minutes later, he had to go again—and every ten to fifteen minutes after that. By 4:00 p.m., his mother was home. The cookies were gone. John was sitting at the kitchen table as his mother walked through the kitchen door. When he said to his mom, "Guess what? I peed forty times today," she had a talk with the babysitter. Next thing he knew, his mother was on the phone with the doctor, and he didn't get to eat dinner. He was lying in the back of his mother's Datsun 240Z hatchback, looking up and out through the window at the blue sky with the fading sun way out over the horizon as he headed toward the children's hospital.

CHILD'S PERSPECTIVE

The child goes from feeling fine to feeling woozy and hollow inside as the day goes on. He can't stop drinking. There is confusion and some fascination (at least for John) with the increase in urination. Fear starts to set in as the adults around him look very serious all of a sudden, whisper to one another so he won't hear their concerns, and/or start panicking. John remembered being pulled by the arm from the house toward the car in a big hurry and being very scared. No one explained what was going on as it was happening—which made it even scarier.

PARENTAL ADVICE

Don't freak out! Calmly, call your child's pediatric doctor, and then take your child to the nearest hospital as soon as possible. Make a concerted effort not to call in front of your child, as John's mother did. He only got half of the conversation, but he clearly saw the fear on his mother's face, which made him fearful too. Your child might be excited or curious about what has been happening to him or her. Don't confuse it for understanding. Depending on the age of your child, he or she may not comprehend what is happening. No matter how much they may act like an adult, remember that they are still children and must be taken care of emotionally. If your child is old enough to understand, you may want to explain that they may be sick before you call their pediatrician. Your child will be very scared. You need to keep calm and focus on comforting your child. When the doctor tells you to head to the hospital, tell your child that you need to go to the hospital to make sure nothing is wrong.

Remember, the doctor has already told you a lot of information. You will be scared yourself, but remain calm. You need to be there for your child. Keep in mind that until you arrive at the hospital, all of the tests have been completed, and the doctor has informed you that your child has diabetes, you simply don't know what is wrong. Don't jump to conclusions that will only make you more scared and upset. Try to get someone to go with you and your child for emotional support—for you. Stay with your child whenever possible. If not, while checking in, have the friend sit with him or her while you do the paperwork. All hospital procedures are different. Some places will not require you to go into the emergency room; others will. Ask the pediatrician when you have him on the phone and get his recommendation on where to go. In some areas, there are special children's hospitals. If possible, go there. If your insurance pays for it or you can afford it, get a private room for your child to avoid any conflicts with other patients.

CLINICAL ADVICE

What *are* the symptoms to look for in children and adults?

Type 1 diabetes, originally called juvenile diabetes, is an autoimmune disorder of the insulin-producing beta cells of the pancreas. It is believed that white blood cells that are used to attack and kill foreign bodies in the bloodstream see the cells that produce insulin as foreign bodies and therefore kill them, permanently destroying them. White blood cells, or leukocytes, are part of the immune system, which defends the human body against both infectious disease and foreign materials. These leukocytes mistake the beta cells for foreign objects and attack them until none are left to produce insulin.

The most important symptom to look out for is *frequent urinations* all day long. As sugar builds in one's blood with no insulin available to unlock the fat cells that store glucose, one's blood sugar rises. It is true that the liver can store and process sugar, but it soon becomes too much to handle. The kidneys can't filter sugar back into the bloodstream. To dilute the sugar, the body draws water from the blood, filling the bladder, which causes frequent urinations. The longer this situation continues, the greater the chance of ketoacidosis. This is a serious condition that can lead to a diabetic coma or even death. It normally takes days to reach this point, and the symptoms are visible much earlier on. Ketoacidosis is the result of very high levels of ketones in your body. Ketones are acids that build up in the bloodstream when one's diabetes is out of control from high blood sugars. Normally people with diabetes test for them often as part of controlling and managing their diabetes.

The next symptom to watch for is *increased levels of thirst*, as your child wants to drink around the clock. The body starts to dehydrate as it reaches a state of ketoacidosis.

Another symptom that can occur is drastic *weight loss* for no apparent reason. Since the sugar/glucose is being urinated out of the body, the body has no source of energy to run on. It starts to break down fat and muscle tissue for energy.

All of these symptoms are followed by *weakness and fatigue*. Insulin is needed to convert glucose into energy for the cells of our body. With glucose remaining unconverted in the bloodstream, the cells begin to starve—causing fatigue.

2

What the "Diabetes Diagnosis" Means

FRIDAY, MAY 27, 1988

On the first morning in Mary's hospital room, she was thinking about her last birthday and how great the cake had tasted and how much fun it had been. She was looking forward to her next party, but she was upset that she would be in the hospital on her birthday. Her mom said that it was going to be all right, that the cake had already been bought.

Mary was in the hospital for two nights and two days. The first night, well, she didn't remember much. Her mom waited in her hospital room that night until her dad arrived. They both were saying that things were going to be all right, but she could see the pain on their faces. She didn't remember much about that evening except that she didn't want her parents to leave.

Her mother came into the room on Saturday morning. She was crying. She grabbed Mary and held her. Mary asked her mom why she was crying, but she never got a response. Later that day, the doctor came in to see her.

Her mother was there when the doctor came in, and he proceeded to inform Mary and her mother that she had diabetes. Mary asked what that was. He said that her body was no longer producing insulin. He also told her that she'd have to take shots of insulin from now on. She was scared, but she asked him how long she'd have to take these shots of insulin (whatever that was). "Will my body ever make insulin again?" she asked. She really didn't understand much of what he was telling her, but she did understand one thing after he answered her question: her body would not produce insulin again—ever. He explained that she'd have to take shots for the rest of her life. A harsh reality to deal with for a soon-to-be seven-year-old. Tomorrow she would be a child pretending to be an adult dealing with an adult problem.

MAN PLANS AND GOD LAUGHS

So here is how the plan was supposed to go: Mary's father was going to give her shots in the morning and evening time, and she was to test her urine for high and low levels of sugar four times daily. She was told to test (under the supervision of an adult) once in the morning, before lunch, before dinner, and before she went to bed. As the doctor laid the plan out, she got more scared of all these things she would have to do. The day before, her biggest worry was that she wouldn't get to play with her Lite-Brite. If her sugar was too high, then the insulin needed to be adjusted, and so on. It was already over her head. Toward the end, the doctor asked for her opinion on how she wanted to manage her sugar levels. At that time, there were two choices. Today children are encouraged to be put on insulin pumps immediately, but they didn't have this choice back then. Mary could either adjust the insulin in accordance with the quantity of food/sugar she was eating at each meal or keep the insulin quantity fixed and weigh the food instead so she would eat the same amount of food for each meal. She picked (and her mother agreed with) the first option. (More on this decision is discussed in the diabetes management styles in the "Clinical Advice" below.)

The doctor asked whether Mary had any questions, and she didn't. Her mother did—lots: What do I do if her sugar is too low, if it's too high, if she wants to ride a bike, if Jupiter and Mars are aligned? You name it, she asked it. The doctor left shortly after, and Mary's father came in later that day. He spent all day practicing giving a shot to an orange. He spent eight hours practicing because she was being released on Sunday, her birthday, he told her. But as her dad told her that he was going to give her the shots, Mary already knew it wasn't going to happen. She didn't remember much more of that day, but she did remember later that night. She had no rules. She could stay up as late as she wanted. She watched movies on TV and ran up and down the hallways, throwing her stuffed animal in the air and catching it. A nurse eventually asked her to go back into her room. She did and watched some more TV until she fell asleep.

CHILD'S PERSPECTIVE
It is very scary for a young child to be alone in a strange place like a hospital. When Mary's mother came in crying, it confused her. After all, she didn't get hurt; Mary did. Mary wanted her mother to stop crying and ask her how she was. She was the sick and hurt one. She asked herself, "Why is Mommy crying, and what is wrong with her?" She worried that if something was wrong with Mommy, who would be there for her? Being told that you have diabetes and that it will be forever is more than scary. You feel alone, confused, angry, and sad and that there is something wrong with you—all at once. The thought that ran through Mary's head that Saturday night was "What did I do wrong to deserve this?" Since she did something wrong, she had to do something right to reverse it—but what was right?

PARENTAL ADVICE
Ask the doctor whether you can stay with your child overnight and, if you can, make sure at least one parent stays (if not both). Make sure that someone brings your child's stuffed animal, wooby, or anything that your child is attached to from his or her bedroom at home, especially if it is something your child sleeps with every night. Remember, children can be very observant. Stress and worry show on people's faces, so even when you tell them that everything will be all right, they may get a mixed message. Better to say what you really know . . . but because you don't really know whether everything will be all right, be honest

but comforting. For example, you could say, "I know you're scared and worried, but whatever happens, we are here for you and you are not alone." Then show it by spending as much time with your child as you can in the first few weeks. This is no time to go to work. Your child needs you now more than ever; whatever else is happening in your life can wait. Your child needs you to be a strong parent. I know you are scared too, but he or she needs you. If you spend this time crying or arguing with everyone and anyone, then your child will feel alone and abandoned. Constant reassurance that children will not face diabetes by themselves is helpful throughout the whole process.

CLINICAL ADVICE

There are several different styles of managing diabetes. Which one is best?

I will do my best to give you the positives and negatives. There are three different types of distinct self-management styles for type 1 diabetes: the methodical style, the adaptive style, and the inadequate style. To help you better understand the three management techniques, we will need to first look at how people with diabetes measure the level of sugar in their blood.

Defining the HbA1c

HbA1c is a measurement of the amount of glycosylated hemoglobin in your blood. Glycosylated hemoglobin is a molecule that attaches to glucose (blood sugar) in red blood cells. The higher the HbA1c you have, the more glucose there is in your blood over a two- to three-month period. For optimum control, the HbA1c test should be taken every three months. The higher your HbA1c levels are, the greater the risk of developing future problems such as heart disease, nerve damage, eye disease, kidney disease, and stroke. If your HbA1c remains high for a long period of time, the risk will increase. When a child or an adult with diabetes maintains healthy, age-appropriate levels of HbA1c, they lower the risk for diabetes-related illness to manifest. For adults, healthy levels are 7 percent or below.

If your child's HbA1c is higher than 8.5 percent, depending on age (set by the American Diabetes Association), then treatment (insulin, quantity of blood tests, etc.), exercise routines, or diet will need to change. A HbA1c level of less than 7 percent means that the blood sugar average is less than 154 mg/dL when you average all the self-monitoring blood glucose tests taken over a three-month period. The lower the average blood sugar level, the higher the risk of having a low blood sugar reaction (less than 70 mg/dL).

On average, the HbA1c level of a person without diabetes will range between 4 and 6 percent. Blood sugars of 70 mg/dL or lower are dangerous and should be avoided. Most doctors I have encountered want your sugar levels to be between 70 and 120 mg/dL. The ADA recommendation is a target area of 70 mg/dL premeal to 130 mg/dL two hours postmeal for adults, with an after-meal peak of 180 mg/dL. The American College of Endocrinology actually has a safer target area of 110 premeal to 140 mg/dL two hours postmeal. This range can relieve emotional stress and pressure for some people with diabetes, as it may be more obtainable. The American Diabetes Association has set age-appropriate levels for HbA1c targets:

1. For children younger than six years old, the target is 8.5 percent.
2. For six- to twelve-year-olds, the target is under 8 percent.
3. For teens (ages thirteen to nineteen), the target is under 7.5 percent.
4. For adults, the target is under 7 percent.

To help simplify the relationship between mg/dL results and HbA1c, see table 2.1, which shows the correlation between HbA1c levels and blood glucose mg/dL as seen on most self-testing instruments. In a later discussion, we'll dig deeper into the relationship between high HbA1c and learning and psychiatric disorders. For now, simply be aware of the healthy levels for the person with diabetes you know and care for.

Table 2.1.

HbA1c	mg/dL	HbA1c	mg/dL	HbA1c	mg/dL
4	68	8	183	12	298
5	97	9	212	13	326
6	126	10	240	14	355
7	154	11	269	15	384

Structured Meal Planning

The first type of meal planning is called the methodical style, in which you create careful meal plans and accurate insulin injections. I like to think of this one as the "cafeteria style" where all meals are portioned and measured. If your child is on a two-hundred-carbohydrate meal plan, each portion size for each meal is measured in grams and weighed on a scale to confirm the resulting carbohydrate intake. Your child's insulin intake is regulated based on the amount of carbohydrates they ingest, so this meal plan ensures that your child eats the same amount of carbohydrates and gets the same amount of insulin for each meal. What is not taken into account is exercise (which burns sugar) or illness (which will lower your metabolism), plus a lot of other factors that can affect blood sugar levels. These are often hidden variables that can disrupt the intended structure of this style of management. This style requires a strict diet, which is particularly hard for adolescents, but some children do very well with the structure. However, no matter how well a child does on it, once they reach adolescence most children start to mismanage their diabetes. Set times, types, and quantities of food on this type of plan leave no room for flexibility if the ice cream truck is parked in front of your house. The methodical style gives great structure and consistency for younger children. However, due to life changes and unpredictability later in life, it is tough to sustain this structure and not realistic to implement it indefinitely.

Balanced Food Planning

The adaptive style is more complex but allows for tighter control, better blood sugars, and more flexibility. So . . . we were saying in the last example that the ice cream truck is parked in front of your house and your child with diabetes hears the bells. This is not a problem for the adaptive style of management; just give a shot of Humalog or other rapid-acting insulin, and it's ice cream for everyone! I have personally used the adaptive style for thirty years. This style works best with an insulin pump. For those manually injecting rapid-acting insulin with a syringe or insulin pen, it may seem a little more daunting, but it can be done and is done by millions of children and adults with diabetes every day. For those not on the pump, a second but long-acting insulin is needed. Long-acting insulin works for twenty-four hours, slowly releasing insulin into the body to cover the amount of insulin needed for proper maintenance.

When one is using long-acting insulin alone, blood sugar stays consistent throughout the day (if other variables don't interfere). This process is similar to an insulin pump that slowly releases insulin into the body all day long. So if your child is on long-acting insulin, then when your child eats, he or she has to give a shot to add more insulin to cover the food. Before insulin became available, the only treatment for diabetes was starvation and exercise. Life expectancy for a person with diabetes before the introduction of insulin was one year, at best. If your child takes no insulin at all, since their body doesn't produce insulin, his or her blood sugar levels will rise even if they don't eat. Therefore, insulin must be provided to the body to regulate these inherently rising levels.

If your child wants to eat, they need to give a shot to counterbalance the food intake. For example, if an individual normally consumes sixty carbohydrates during an average dinner meal on rotisserie chicken

night—leg and thigh combo with a serving of rice and some veg-
etables—they may, depending on their insulin-to-carbohydrate ratio
(provided by their endocrinologist or a CDE), need to give one unit of
Humalog for each ten grams of carbohydrates, which comes to six units
of rapid-acting insulin for this meal.

However, today your Great Aunt Joanne brought over her famous
cheesecake for dessert, and you want a piece. No problem. If you know
before eating it that you'll need to give more rapid-acting insulin, depending on how many carbohydrates that big piece of that yummy
cheesecake you want to eat has in it, instead of the regular six units
you'd normally take before a sixty-carbohydrate dinner, you may have
to give an additional four units (if the cheesecake has forty carbohydrates in it). Units vary depending on the individual; see your endocrinologist to learn your personal "insulin-to-carbohydrate" ratio.

If Great Aunt Joanne drops by unexpectedly after dinner with the
cheesecake, then you will have to take another shot of four units or
administer (bolus) another four units of insulin via your pump and enjoy. If employing this style, it is important to test blood sugars multiple
times a day to check for high or low blood sugars and then make the
necessary adjustments as prescribed by your endocrinologist or certified diabetes educator.

If on Monday, Wednesday, and Friday your child plays basketball
after school, then either a reduction of insulin or a snack before playing will keep his sugar levels in balance. During sports or any type of
exercise, it is important that rapid-acting glucose be available in case
of a reaction. If your child is struggling to eat the rapid-acting glucose,
then four ounces of orange juice or hard candies like Life Savers® or rock
candy will give the child a little sense of normalcy. (Word of caution:
Avoid chocolate and other fatty treats, as they take too long to work.)

The adaptive style of management allows for your child to have a
piece of cake at a birthday party and other special events. I am not saying that the child should be given carte blanche to eat what they want,
but one or two times a week won't hurt, considering that it will reduce
their desire to cheat because they know that, when it counts, they will

be able to get a Mister Softee with the rest of the neighborhood children. This style keeps the same type of blood sugar control and HbA1c levels as the methodical style, but it has been proven to be more flexible in the wake of changes in the individual's lifestyle and to satisfy the need for autonomy throughout adolescence and on.

"Eat What You Want" Food Planning

The third self-management technique is called the "inadequate style" with moderate rates of self-care adjustments. Research has shown that the previous two styles we discussed have an HbA1c of 8 percent, which is okay. The inadequate style has an average of 9.6 percent. This style puts children at risk for future health-related problems, including psychiatric issues, by interfering with the healthy development of the brain. In this style, there is no active focus on health-related activities that are needed to maintain proper HbA1c levels like exercise, insulin, or food management. Instead, children and their families make minimal self-care adjustments.

The more flexible and adjustable one's treatment is, the better control a child has. Good control creates physical and mental health. It is my feeling that the HbA1c levels are a little high in this style, considering the multiple risks these can cause to the development of the brain. However, it is very important to consult with a pediatric endocrinologist or a certified diabetes educator before making any changes to your child's diabetes management.

Impulsive Experimentation

The first time I was on Lantus, I didn't eat all day (not recommended) to see the effect. I started around 120 mg/dL and ended the day at the same level. After ten blood checks, nothing changed. I was excited about the prospect of one less variable to control for. For many years, I have used a combination of Lantus and Humalog to control my diabetes. Now I am on the pump, and every day I am excited, as it has taken more variables away and reduced my already good HbA1c by close to 1 percent.

3

Managing My First Shot and My Family

SUNDAY, SEPTEMBER 18, 1977

I woke up the morning of my sixth birthday thinking, "Just leave me alone!" There were balloons and flowers strewn throughout my room amid the get-well cards. My mother and father, a nurse, and a doctor were in the room. The doctor told me that it was time for breakfast, but before I could eat, I would need to be given a shot. The nurse gave the shot to my father, and they approached my bed together. My dad was being directed by the nurse to give me the shot, just like they had practiced. I told her I would not take it. Everyone proceeded to tell me all the reasons why I had to take the shot, with explanation after explanation. After about twenty minutes of back and forth, a very pissed-off nurse finally said the right thing: "Why don't you want to take the shot?" (Grownups can be so stupid around kids. They treat children as if they don't know what is best for themselves when they do. Ironically, they do let their kids make decisions at times when they actually don't know what is best for them. You may have seen it when the parent tells the child they can eat whatever they want.) At this point, I was frustrated and shouted at her, "I want to give it!" A shocked nurse asked, "Why?" I replied, "The doctor told me that I was going to have this my whole life. Right?" She said, "Yes." I replied, "I need to do this at some point, so why not now?" She listened to me and seemed to understand my point, so she let me do it.

The nurse showed me first how to hold the syringe. She then helped me to squeeze the muscle and jab the needle into it. There were mixed reactions from everyone, and the whole hospital was talking about it. My mother looked happy and proud. My father looked relieved and pissed at the same time. (I would be too if I had spent eight hours sticking an orange with a syringe.) The doctor said, "What a brave child," and shook my hand. The nurse told the whole nursing staff. She kind of had to because they just happened to come by to talk. I was relieved, scared, and proud of myself, all at the same time.

It was 1:00 p.m. the following day, and we were preparing to leave the hospital. My mom asked whether I was ready to leave, and I said yes, but I actually wanted to stay. I was scared of doing all this by myself, but I knew I had to, so we left. In the car on the ride home, I noticed a big fruit basket in the back of the car. I asked, "Mom, what is the big basket of fruit for?" She said, "It is for your birthday party. Now that you are a diabetic, you can't have cake, so this is just as good." A few moments went by. Then I sadly said, "But you promised me chocolate cake!" Her response was "Well, I know I did. Thing are going to have to be different from now on. You are not allowed to have cake or anything with sugar in it." I repeated, "But you promised!" My mom replied, "Well, you can't have it, and that's it!" I was like most kids after their parent lies to them, and I continued to argue: "But I want it. Everyone else gets to." My mom was getting upset, and she told me, "The doctor said no sweets, so no sweets!" I cried the rest of the way home. I felt like it was the worst day of my life. I didn't feel different and I was still me, so why was I was labeled different?

I don't remember much of the party that year. I do remember feeling more alone than I ever did, even around my friends. From then on, I still didn't feel different, but people treated me differently. I was now a child with diabetes, and no longer just an innocent child.

My dad moved out a year after I was diagnosed, to the day. The truth was that things at home were not going as well as I am sure my parents envisioned when they decided to get married. Eventually they got divorced, when I was about eight years old. I felt it was my fault because I got diabetes.

CHILD'S PERSPECTIVE

Diabetes is scary, and it is even scarier to take your first injection. No matter how grown up children may behave, the reality is that they are frightened. In truth, I am not sure whether my mother or father tried to console me during my stay in the hospital. I'm not even sure they knew how. Being in the hospital was terrifying for all of us. It can be very confusing with nurses and doctors coming in and out of your room all the time and no one telling you what is going on. It is mysterious and intimidating. This is true for most children, and most adults, who are lying in a hospital bed. I felt like everything was spinning out of control.

I, like most children, was very upset, worried, and confused by my experience at the hospital in general. I did not have the emotional awareness or the skills to verbalize it. Worst of all, I felt angry toward my parents for not protecting me. Like many children, I had intense emotions about my stay at the hospital. I went from feeling safe and secure at home to what I perceived as a frightening and crazy world where I was constantly poked and prodded, over and over again. I wanted to be comforted and feel supported; instead, I felt alone in a cold hospital room. I did not want to feel this way, but I could not explain my feelings at that time. I did not know how to say I felt alone. Unfortunately, that was exactly how I felt—I felt alone with this illness. Toward the end of my stay at the hospital, I felt better, but I was still terrified. I was no longer scared of being in the hospital, but I was afraid to leave. I did not want to go home where there would be no nurses or doctors to help me. I felt as though I had to rely on myself, and if I messed up, I could die. It was scary to leave the support of the doctors and nurses.

As I was leaving the hospital, I thought to myself, "Who will take care of me now?!" The first time I truly felt different was on the drive home. It is different for each child. I felt sad, but I did not know why. It was not until much later in life that I realized the massive loss that happened

that day on the drive home. I lost my freedom as well as my ability to
feel safe in the world, and there was no way to get my old life back.

PARENTAL ADVICE

Be aware that not all children show emotion the way a parent expects
them to. I didn't. Diabetes is a lifelong disorder. It is difficult to accept
that you even have it at first. I myself had a wide range of emotions,
including anger, sadness, and frustration, just to name a few. No matter how I felt in the moment or around the diabetes, I felt I could not
show it when others were around. I did not want to worry my parents,
so I acted strong and pretended that I was able to take care of myself in
an effort to protect them. What I did not know how to do was protect
myself from my fears and ask for support.

While your child may be able to give himself or herself an injection,
bolus on their own, or test their own blood sugar at a very early age, it
is important to remember that he or she is still a child. He or she will
need your help, not just in managing his or her diabetes but also with
understanding his or her feelings.

Every child is different. Regardless of what age yours is, active parental involvement will be needed. Whether your child says it or not,
he or she will need your emotional support. It is difficult—in fact, next
to impossible—for a young child to live with diabetes alone, to make
lifestyle adjustments, to manage his or her own blood sugars, or to cope
with the emotional rollercoaster ride that is diabetes.

Depending on age, there is only so much you will be able to do to
help your child. Make sure there is open communication about feelings.
Let your child know that he or she is not alone and that you will help
him or her through this process. Do not try to control him or her or tell
your child how to feel. The goal is for your child to feel that he or she
has a team and that everyone's input matters, including his or her own.

It is important to remember that your child needs to feel in control.
Based on his or her age, your child needs to be consulted and given the
opportunity to express how he or she wants to handle his or her diabetes.

You also need to guide and support them with making healthy choices. Take the time to work with them to understand the disorder, learn about it together, and teach them how to make better choices for themselves (as age appropriate). Children need to *feel* that they have an equal say in managing their diabetes, even if they are at an age when you are making 95 percent of the choices. Look for places they can participate, even if it is just placing a test strip in the meter or picking the color of the carrying case for their pump.

It is very scary not just for the child but also for the parent. Sometimes, as parents, we become overprotective. It is important not to do this, as a little cake won't do permanent damage to someone with diabetes when extra insulin is given to adjust accordingly for it. The emotional impact of being overprotective or strict can have a longer-lasting impact. My mother was technically correct in her decision to choose fruit instead of cake. When managing diabetes, fruit is easier to break down and will not impact blood sugar levels as much as cake would. She took care of the diabetes management but forgot to incorporate the fact that I was a six-year-old child into her decision-making process. It is essential to personalize diabetes management and adjust it to your child, unless your child prefers fruit to cake. It is more effective to slowly change your child's diet instead of imposing what may feel like a sudden shift and potentially a penalty. The child may feel confused and hurt and attempt to figure out what he or she did to deserve such treatment. A better choice would be to still have cake, but maybe a smaller piece would suffice.

When a person is worried or scared, it is difficult to think clearly. My mother's feelings got in the way of her choices around my sixth birthday party. In the present moment, it is difficult to make these decisions and remember to also address your child to find out his or her input about the changes being made. It is important to communicate clearly with your child around decisions that will affect him or her. There are a couple of things that would have lessened the impact of my mother's decision for me: if we had discussed ahead of time how I would feel about having to have fruit for my birthday instead of cake, and if she had given me prior notification of the change before I got in the car and saw the fruit basket. If that discussion had happened first, I still would not have been happy about it, but I would have felt like I was part of the decision-making process. Luckily, there are ways to adjust for cake in diabetes management, like reducing the portion of cake while adjusting your child's insulin bolus to match the carbs.

Interestingly enough, the more fat there is in the treat, the harder it is for the body to convert it to glucose, which allows rapid-acting insulin to be more efficient. Basically, the higher the fat content, the lower insulin resistance becomes, reducing the impact food has on blood sugar levels.

CLINICAL ADVICE

Age-Appropriate Management of Diabetes

Table 3.1.

Age	Food	Insulin	Testing	Psychological
4–5	Your child knows what foods he/she likes and dislikes.	Can tell where the injection should be injected and use alcohol swab on their skin to prepare for the injection.	Collects his or her own urine for ketone testing. S/he can turn on the meter and help with recording.	Identifies with "good" and "bad." Using these words, a child this age may think she is bad if the test results are labeled as "bad."
6–7	Children begin to understand carbohydrates. They know which foods to limit.	Can help with other aspects of insulin delivery, beyond using alcohol swabs. Can enter insulin units into a pump.	When testing their own blood sugar levels, they can prick their finger.	They need reminders to check their blood sugar and urine for ketones. They should be supervised when testing blood and urine.

Age	Food	Insulin	Testing	Psychological
8–10	Can select their food and may know how to adjust insulin with supervision.	They may draw up their own shots or enter units of bolus with supervision, depending on individual ability.	They can keep records of blood sugar and do their own blood sugar tests with supervision.	Need reminders and understand only the immediate consequences of diabetes.
11–13	Can start using a search engine to look up carb amounts to assist with carb counting.	They can measure and inject or bolus own insulin without reminders or supervision.	Can see blood test results forming a pattern with some supervision.	May be rebellious. Concerned less with controlling diabetes and more with fitting in.
14+	They may start eating out with friends and not adjust for food when with their friends.	If they haven't already started, they can adjust, mix insulin, or reduce basal rate when needed.	May begin using test results to adjust insulin. Inform them to adjust for food, even with friends.	Knows short- and long-term consequences. Independence is important. Needs to know support is at home if needed.

Note: This chart is a guide to age-appropriate self-care. Some children are able to do more or less, depending on their level of individual capability.

Emotional Needs

There are several emotions that form around the diagnosis of diabetes and living with it that parents need to be aware of: grief, anger, depression, fear, guilt, and denial. Normally, your children may have many of these feelings. You and other members of the family may feel them too. The sooner you and your child come to accept the diagnosis and move away from self-blame, the happier the family will be and the better controlled the child's condition will become.

Grief

Grief is typically known as the sadness that occurs after the loss of a loved one. It can also happen after any loss, especially if the person places a high value on the lost person, place, or thing. In my case, it was the end of a carefree lifestyle, a life I had known that didn't involve managing chronic illness.

Parents may grieve the loss of "the healthy child." Typically, the sooner the parents accept that they cannot protect their child from everything, the sooner the healing process can begin. The parents may grieve their loss of lifestyle too, as they are forced to change many things, from the time for dinner to what the family eats to taking on other responsibilities that come with managing their child's diabetes.

Loss of control can cause a parent or child to grieve. Many small things happen that are a part of the lifestyle change, including having to go back home to get forgotten diabetes supplies after driving an hour to a friend's house for dinner. A low blood sugar reaction in their child can take away the parents' plans and control, causing the parent watching the child to change his or her plans in order to help the child raise his or her blood sugar back to normal. Sometimes this may require a trip to the hospital. These and other events that come with diabetes can perpetuate the feeling of grief. Being flexible and accepting of the changes that come with diabetes, along with time, will reduce one's grief. Open discussion around the loss as a family can help as well. In an effort to help the children in your family, let them know that you are there for them and encourage talking about how they feel. Then pay attention and listen. Talk therapy can also help an individual or family come to acceptance.

Anger

Anger is a normal part of life. Unfortunately for the child with diabetes, there is more than enough to share. I was angry with both of my parents for not protecting me and for allowing me to get diabetes. Most people displace anger onto others who are not at fault. It is also easy for anger at oneself to quickly turn into depression. Some people direct their anger appropriately, talk about it effectively, and eventually accept that they have diabetes, which reduces their anger. Children with diabetes may inappropriately become angry at their friends, siblings, and you, the parent, instead of the illness. This is often too hard for children to understand, especially young children. Parents can also fall into this trap of getting angry at themselves and, inadvertently, at others. They get mad at themselves for not protecting their child from such a disorder (as if they could) as well as their spouse, and even at the doctor, instead of coming to the realization that no one is at fault. It is just part of life. *Diabetes just happens.*

Depression

Depression doesn't need to be a part of everyone's life, but many people go through it from time to time. Anger turned inward is how most look at it, but with diabetes it usually revolves around self-blame and negative self-talk. Your child may feel hopeless, sad without being able to express it in a verbal manner, or may tell you that his or her life is now ruined because of diabetes. Self-blame and negative self-talk also occur in the parents who feel, as most parents do, that they are the protectors of their children. Unfortunately, as hard as we try, we cannot always protect our children from everything and have to accept that it is not our fault when it comes to diabetes. You may find yourself more emotional than normal and dwelling on negative thoughts around your child's future. Do your best to stay away from these types of thoughts. There is nothing that could have been done to prevent the onset of diabetes. Stay positive and enjoy your time with your child. They can have a long, productive, and happy life. Remember, children will watch you to see how you choose to handle their diagnosis of diabetes. The more positive you are, the better the example you will set for your child.

Fear

Fear is a natural part of life. As living creatures, humans fear different things. Some fear the unknown. Some fear change, and some fear everything. Fear is a powerful emotion and is needed for survival. It helps you to decide whether to fight or run. Too much fear, and you may run and hide from everything; too little fear, and you may walk through the world with blinders on, putting yourself at great risk of mental and physical harm. Fear is needed. It makes us feel cautious when encountering certain or possible dangers. It raises our awareness so we pay closer attention to what is occurring and what is around us. It causes a person to look both ways before crossing the street. Fear of hurting another can help motivate us to be honest with those we love. It can also prevent us from being honest when we think that the truth may hurt the one we love. Fear can keep us frozen or stuck in one place. For example, when in an abusive relationship, the fear of leaving a known environment to venture forth into the unknown world alone can keep a person from doing what is right for him or her. A certain amount of fear is healthy, but too much or too little can cause you great harm.

Fear comes in many forms. For children with diabetes, it can get very complicated to manage. Some children may fear that they won't fit in with others. Where children with diabetes are concerned, not being accepted is a fear that has the potential to be very real. For example, being treated differently by adults at school and needing accommodations makes them stand out from their peers, thereby reducing their ability to fit in. The fear of having a hypoglycemic reaction (low blood sugar) may cause a child to eat more food in an effort to keep his or her blood sugars high. Over time, this puts these children at risk for developmental issues that can impact the development of their brains. They may fear dying early or losing a leg to gangrene. After all, they can read about these side effects of diabetes on the internet. You cannot hide this information from them. This may lead your child to work harder in managing his or her diabetes. Unfortunately, when the child exerts extremely tight control over their diabetes, it puts them at greater risk for hypoglycemia (low blood sugar). The fear these children have of potentially disappointing their parents or not living up to their expectations may motivate them to keep their diabetes under better control. However, using fear to motivate a child will last only so long. Eventually your child will need to find positive motivators to maintain healthy management in the long run.

Most unhealthy, irrational fear can be summed up in the acronym FEAR—False Evidence Appearing Real. For example, very few people who maintain good management of their type 1 diabetes lose their legs or eyesight anymore. Believing you will if you aren't in perfect control is False Evidence Appearing Real.

When fear is irrational, it causes anxiety. Like fear, anxiety is good in proper moderation, but too much of it, and you won't function properly or think clearly. Conversely, too little of it, and you will have no motivation. Parents tend to have extremely high levels of anxiety around their child's diabetes as a result of self-blame and the fear that if they make a mistake in treating their child's diabetes, they might hurt or kill their child. This line of thinking is also False Evidence Appearing Real. It can cause you to feel overwhelmed and make it ten times harder to be there and present for your child. If you work together as a team with your child, allow your child to discuss problems with you about the diabetes, and make concessions regarding your child's problems or fears, then your child will be fine. You can only do what you and your child are capable of. There is no model child with diabetes, and you didn't cause your child to have diabetes. *It just happened.*

Guilt

Guilt is also part of being human, but it is part of everyday life for some children living with diabetes and their parents. "I cheated on my diet. I should have known better. I am so stupid for eating that piece of cake at my friend's birthday party. I am so stupid!" It is difficult when everyone around you can eat whatever he or she wants. The pressure to fit in may have caused a slip like this, but inevitably guilt follows; however, it doesn't have to. We blame ourselves because we tend to create higher standards for ourselves than we can reach. For children, it is the standards their parents set that impact how they view their actions.

It is okay to be human. We are imperfect beings driven to strive for perfection. No matter how hard you try, no one is perfect. A parent should respond to a child the first time something like this happens with "It's okay. I don't expect you to be perfect. As long as you try your best, I am proud of you. Let's look at how you can fit in with your friends and still have good blood sugars at the same time."

Children may feel responsible for the burden they believe their diabetes is putting on their families, or they may feel that it is their fault that they got diabetes in the first place. Having several discussions about how the diabetes is not a burden, that the family supports the child out of love, and that it is not their fault that they got diabetes is very beneficial for the child. When having these discussions with your child, please keep this in mind: *"It is not your fault either!"* Genetics have been passed down for thousands of years, and you can not control that. *It just happens.*

Remind yourself that every time you start to self-blame, you are thinking irrationally, and that the truth is there are some things that no one has control over—and this is one of them. Don't blame yourself for not recognizing that your child had a problem earlier because that would be irrational thinking as well. Would you blame yourself if you failed to be hired as the pitcher of the New York Yankees if you had never played baseball in your life? No, you wouldn't. The same is true of diabetes. Until you or your child has it, you wouldn't know what to look for.

Denial

Denial is most commonly thought of when people discuss addiction. For example, a person sits in a bar and drinks for hours every Friday night after work. Sometimes his coworkers come, but if not, he drinks alone and gets home around 4:00 a.m. on Saturday morning. Over the course of one evening, he consumes fifteen beers and shots of vodka. He leaves the bar, gets in a cab, and goes home. He has a blood alcohol content (BAC) of 4 percent, or .4. The legal limit in most states is under .05 to drive. He is at eight times the legal limit. He keeps a monthly tab at the bar. All his friends and coworkers have had discussions with him about his drinking problem. Every Saturday afternoon when he wakes up, he has a hangover (the equivalent of withdrawal). His wife is leaving him because he is never home for her or the kids and they can't pay the rent. If you asked him whether he thought he was drinking too much or called him an alcoholic, he would simply say that he just drinks a few after work to blow off some steam. In this scenario, he would be categorized as being in denial.

Denial comes in many forms. With diabetes, your child may similarly say that he or she doesn't have diabetes or that it will just go away on its own. She or he may not take (or try to get out of taking) insulin. Your child may eat poorly, such as junk food not in the plan or things like candy, and then try to get out of testing their blood. When forced, he or she may go into the bathroom unobserved and lie about the results from testing it. Believe me, I know. Some of these things are things I did on a regular basis during my first few years with diabetes.

My mother also had trouble with grieving and accepting that I had diabetes. She blamed herself for my illness, which was out of both of our control. Because my mother didn't have the same resources that parents have today, such as seeing a psychotherapist to work through her feelings of loss and grief, it took her twenty-five years to accept that I had diabetes and it wasn't her fault. *It just happened.*

It is normal for your child and you as the parent to feel the above emotions, and it can be very confusing. Understanding the physical and emotional aspects of living with diabetes will help reduce these negative feelings. No one is at fault—no one. *It just happens.*

4

What Going Back to School Means

MONDAY, OCTOBER 22, 1979

"Because everyone thinks they know what's best for me, no one ever asks. I am returning to school tomorrow after being in the hospital for several days. My birthday was ruined. No cake. No ice cream. This is when it begins—the looks, the stares I don't fully understand, and wondering whether my school friends can understand something I don't."

Nathan was nine years old when he was diagnosed with diabetes. He was only in school for about five weeks before he left for the hospital. It has been a few days since then, but fourth grade wasn't great to begin with—and now this. He guessed things would be okay tomorrow. He would just close his eyes, and it would all be better when he woke up tomorrow. Maybe the diabetes would be gone and nothing would have changed. As Nathan drifted off, he remembered being back in the hospital and how scared he was.

It's early in the morning. Since nothing had changed, he was still a child with diabetes, which meant more problems. "I don't feel so hot," he said to himself. Nathan tested his urine, and the strip changed to brown. His blood sugar was high again. He shrugged his shoulders, got ready for school, and went downstairs. He saw his dad and heard him cursing to himself. He had already drawn the shot. Darn. "Well, I'm not going to be the one to tell him my blood sugar is high," he said to himself, not after what happened when he had to draw his shot a second time yesterday.

Before dinner the previous night, his father had already drawn his shot and Nathan had not tested his blood sugar yet. His father got angry with him because he had to redraw the shot when Nathan told him what his blood sugar level was. His dad asked whether Nathan had tested his sugar this morning. Nathan said he did, and it was light blue—normal. He had school to go to and he didn't want to be yelled at again. He thought, "It will be fine 'til I get home." He remembered how angry his father had been with him the last time his results were high, so Nathan ate breakfast and headed to the bus stop in front of his house. Very convenient, don't you think?

Nathan's mother stopped him and said, "I am taking you to school." Nathan replied, "But I want to go on the school bus." He wanted to be with his friends on the bus. "Don't worry. You will be taking it home, and you will see your friends then. Now come on, I don't want you to be late. The bus isn't coming. I canceled the bus for the rest of the year, so stop this nonsense!" Begrudgingly, Nathan went with his mom, still upset about the bus as well as no cake, no ice cream, and no candy on his birthday. He wondered, "What am I going to tell the kids on the bus about why I can't take the bus in the mornings? That can wait. I have more pressing issues at the moment."

Nathan was quiet for most of the ride. Everything was changing for the worse. Halfway through, he had to go to the bathroom. His *real* pressing issue! He waited for what seemed like hours, but it was actually ten minutes in adult time. Now Nathan was in pain. He had to pee so badly and felt that peeing his pants, something he hadn't done in years, would be the icing on the cake. He said goodbye to his mom and started sprinting into school, right into the bathroom. Ah, relief! "It was the best pee of my life." No, I am not kidding. That was what Nathan said, that it was the best all-time pee ever, over a good minute with heavy stream. He said, "If it was winter, I could write my name and several others in the snow."

Nathan was late for class his first day back. Nathan walked into class, hoping to slip in quietly. Talking to himself, he said, "Did I just hear my name called?" He turned around and Mrs. Jones, his teacher, was calling his name. "Nathan, Nathan, Nathan! Glad to see you finally made it to class." Nathan thought, "Is she really calling me out in front of the whole class?" Nathan responded with "UH?" Mrs. Jones followed up with "I was worried about you. Glad to see you are back in one piece." Woo, dodged the bullet that time. Class went on as normal, but he had to ask permission to go to the bathroom halfway through. This was not a problem for the teacher, but it was definitely one for Nathan. After class, he should have gone to the bathroom, but he didn't, so Nathan had to ask the art teacher for permission to go to the bathroom. Not a problem there either. He guessed that he shouldn't have gone to the water fountain on the way to art class. He didn't remember much of that school day, but he did know that he had to keep going to the bathroom during classes. He did remember the bus ride home. It was a long one.

School ended, and it was now time for Nathan to go home. He went to the front of the bus. The bus was more like a large van painted yellow with the school's name written on the side. The van/bus had maybe four rows of bench-type seating and two bucket seats in the front for the driver and one other person. As Nathan waited for the other students to arrive at the bus, he kept trying to come up with excuses as to why he would not be riding the bus in the morning anymore. Nathan's skills for lying had not fully developed as of yet, so, with eyes to the ground, he said to his friends, "My mother won't let me take the bus in the morning anymore."

Nathan didn't know the reason his mom canceled the bus. She didn't really tell him why. She only told him that he wouldn't be taking the bus in the morning. When the other kids asked why, he couldn't think of anything good to say, so Nathan told the other children that he couldn't go to school by bus because he had diabetes. Lucky for him, the bus driver arrived and said, "All aboard." Everyone got on the bus. Nathan sat in the second-to-last bench by the window. It was a beautiful day to ride the bus. The sky was blue, and you could smell the honeysuckles that grew on the side of the school's driveway.

Nathan didn't talk much normally. On the bus, he had a few friends. They didn't say much to him that trip, but he believed that they just didn't know what to say. Nathan was happy about that, as he didn't know what to say either. "I had a really good friend, Neil, who rode the bus I took and who always sat with me. I stared out the window for most of the ride. I felt that my friends were judging me for being different. About halfway through the ride, Neil tapped me on the shoulder and asked if I wanted a piece of Bazooka Joe bubble gum. It always came wrapped in a comic strip. We both read ours out loud to each other. We both laughed and talked about how funny those comic strips were, and we reminisced about the past ones we got." According to Nathan, this was also the friend who introduced him to Big League Chew bubble gum. He loved it because it was like the chewing tobacco that the baseball players used, but it was gum. He said, "Like chewing tobacco, how awesome is that!" However, Nathan had overlooked the fact that the gum he was chewing was full of sugar. Once he stopped laughing, he noticed that some of the other kids on the bus were looking at him. Nathan knew he shouldn't have told them about his diabetes. He thought to himself, "Damn it! I am so stupid. Why did I tell them? I could have just played dumb." Nathan's friend turned to him and said, "Never mind them. They are just jealous of us." Nathan tried to smile at him, but his friend knew he didn't buy that. A minute later, they were at Neil's bus stop, and he got off the bus. "Bye, Nathan! I will see you tomorrow." "Okay, Neil. See you tomorrow!" He then, all of a sudden, realized that he had to pee again. He told himself, "We will be home in a few moments, so just hold it." He repeated it to himself a couple of times, but it was too late. It came on so strong that he had to just surrender and take a leak on the bus.

So, Nathan gave in and peed his pants. He didn't know what he was going to do next. He said to himself, "Okay. This is the plan. The two kids behind you in the back row will get off next. They are the only ones sitting in the last row. You will pray that no one notices. After they get off, go into the back seat and hide 'til the bus gets to your stop." They got off the bus. "Go now, while you have the chance!" He switched seats. About two minutes later, the bus was at his home. He flew out of the bus and ran into his house. As Nathan got to his house, he started to cry. "Why me? Why?" As he walked in through the front door sobbing, he heard the door shut behind him as he fell to the floor and cried in the fetal position for almost half an hour. Nathan thought, "Oh my God!" His mom was going to be home in an hour and a half. He wondered whether the bus driver knew and whether he was calling his mom. He thought, "Okay. Stop it, Nathan. Pull yourself together and think. You can do this."

He got up off the floor and headed upstairs. Nathan put his backpack on his bed, changed into a fresh pair of clothes, and sat down on the bed. After a few minutes, he realized what he had to do. He took the pants and washed them in the sink with dish soap. When he was confident that they were clean, he took them into the basement and threw them into the dryer. Then he went back upstairs. He figured that the underpants could be thrown out because he didn't think his mother would notice one pair of underwear missing. Nathan put them in a plastic bag. That way, the smell wouldn't be noticed. Then he walked out the kitchen door and down the four cement steps toward the garage door. When he got to the garage door, he opened it by himself. To the left as he entered, he saw his banana seat bike, but right next to the door, up against one of the garage walls, were two huge, gray trash cans with lids on them. He was hoping that there was already a kitchen trash bag in it so he had somewhere to conceal the plastic bag with the underpants in it. Nathan opened the lid, and there it was—his salvation: a partially filled, large, black plastic trash bag. He opened the trash bag and put the plastic bag with his soiled underwear in it. He then closed it up. He smiled as he put the cover back on the trash can and felt a sigh of relief. He thought to himself, "If the sock gnomes can steal our socks while we sleep, why not underwear? That is my story, and I am sticking to it," should his mom notice that the pair of underwear was missing. (A few years later, he learned those socks ended up trapped in the dryer's lint filter.)

Nathan went back into the house and down the flight of stairs to the basement to check on his pants. They weren't dry yet, and that could be a problem. He was wearing blue pants now, but he had gone to school wearing brown ones. If his mother came home before the brown ones were dry, the whole "Operation Pee Pants" would be a failure because his mother might notice. It was now about 4:00 p.m., and Nathan's mom would arrive between 4:30 and 5:00.

Nathan's basement was partly finished. Baseboard heaters ran along the bottom of the fake wood walls, very 1970s. The floor in the laundry room was cement, but the rest of the basement was 12-inch-by-12-inch light greenish-yellow tiles with a flower pattern on them. The only furniture was a full, wooden bar with stools that you passed on the way to the laundry room. Nathan left the laundry room and went upstairs to look out the window for his mom. Every five minutes, he would run down to check on the pants. It was like waiting for a pot of water to boil. On his third trip past the bar, he was craving something sweet. He went behind the bar to look for something good. He saw a powdered martini mix for all different flavors. Nathan tried the lemon one first. He figured that he would try the others on another day. He ripped open the package. As the flavored powdered sugar hit his tongue, he felt so relaxed. It tasted soooooooo good. He crumpled the paper packet up and put it into his pocket, making sure that he threw it away in the kitchen trash. He had learned that when discarding things like candy wrappers in the trash, you needed to make sure that you had other trash to cover up the evidence. All of a sudden, Nathan realized it was twenty minutes later. He ran to the dryer, pulled his blue pants off, and put on the almost dry pair of brown corduroy pants. Nathan hated those pants. As he threw the blue ones in the hamper, he heard his mom's car door close. Nathan ran back upstairs, turned the TV on, fell into the couch, and said hello to his mom as she walked through the kitchen door. She asked him how his day was, and he simply said, "Fine," and went back to watching TV. No one ever found out, and this was just one of many incidences.

TUESDAY, OCTOBER 23, 1979
When Nathan woke up the next morning, his blood sugar was high. The strip had changed to brown again. He hoped that his dad hadn't drawn the shot yet, before he could tell him, but he had. He was going to be honest and tell him—better than going through that again. Nathan told him, and he could swear he heard his father say under his breath that he didn't have time for this. His father drew up another shot with more insulin; then he left for work, complaining about being late. Nathan knew then that this wasn't going to get better.

The ride with his mom to school was better. He made it through first period before having to go to the bathroom. During the middle of art class, he had to pee again. He held it and rushed to the bathroom between periods. It was starting again. Nathan started to cry in the bathroom so no one could see, and he was happy that he was alone. He was late getting to his next class, but he didn't care anymore. Nathan was preoccupied with his thoughts about how this was going to be the rest of his life. The rest of the day went pretty much like the day before. He remembers being in the bathroom more than class. He started to go to the bathroom between periods, even if he didn't feel like he had to urinate, as a preemptive attempt to not leave during class. Only once that day did he have to urinate during class. This time, before going on the bus, he waited until the last minute to use the bathroom.

The bus ride home was different this time. Nathan headed right for the back seat, and the two kids who were there yesterday sat down next to him. Neil got on and asked him why he was not sitting in their usual spot. Nathan said he just wanted to ride in the back from now on. Neil shrugged his shoulders and said, "Tell me next time," as he sat down in the row in front of Nathan. Neil didn't look happy, but if he told him what was going on, he would think Nathan was weird. Nathan thought he might even end their friendship, and Neil was one of his only friends. Nathan kept wanting to talk to Neil, but he sat quietly instead and looked out the window. When the bus got to his stop, Neil got off and said, "If you want, we can both sit in the back tomorrow." Nathan responded with "Okay" and that he would see him in school tomorrow. That was a relief! He had already peed his pants halfway through the trip home, but he played it cool. He left the school bus in less of a rush, looking behind him at his seat to see whether it had gone through his pants. Luckily, it hadn't.

When he was safely inside his house, Nathan went upstairs and calmly put his backpack on his bed. He again changed into a fresh pair of clothes, just like yesterday. There was no time to waste. He immediately started with what he had dubbed "Operation Pee Pants" the day before. Since he had more time today, he washed his pants and underwear in the washing machine. He put some detergent in with them and then started the machine. When the washer was done, he threw them into the dryer. No sock gnomes would be stealing his underwear this time.

After he left the laundry room, Nathan went upstairs and watched some afternoon cartoons. He went down once to check on the pants. Then he went behind the bar again to look for the powdered martini mix. He went for the lemon-flavored packet again, ripping the package open and pouring it into his mouth, thinking how good it was. He went back upstairs and watched more cartoons for another twenty minutes. Then he got his pants and went back to the couch. Ten minutes later, Nathan's mom walked through the kitchen door. She asked him how his day was. He said that it was fine and went back to watching TV. This was a routine that happened way too often from then on, for his taste.

WEDNESDAY, OCTOBER 24, 1979

You are not going to believe this, but Nathan woke up this morning and his urine tested green, in the midrange—not normal but just above normal. Today he felt different as he awoke. He got up and started getting ready for school. As he headed into the kitchen, he noticed that his dad was already gone. His shot was already made, and his dad had left for work. Nathan's choice was made for him, but he didn't have much to tell his father today. School was better for Nathan. He was in a better mood, and he only had to urinate four times, instead of seven times or more. He was getting into a routine of using the bathroom to urinate during the five-minute breaks between classes. If he couldn't pee, he didn't force it. He also made sure he went to the bathroom before getting onto the bus to go home.

Nathan was feeling better, but he was worried about the bus. He got on and got the back seat. Neil followed right behind, sitting next to him. They talked about comic books and what they were going to do over the weekend. Neil invited Nathan over to his house to play on Saturday. Neil said that his brother would be there, but they could just ignore him. Nathan smiled and thanked him. Before Nathan knew it, he had gotten off the bus with dry pants for a change. He didn't know what tomorrow would bring, but for today, he was happy.

SATURDAY, OCTOBER 27, 1979

The rest of his week was about the same as Monday and Tuesday. He went to school with his mom in the morning and found that taking the bus on the way home was continually a challenge. On Thursday, Nathan didn't make it home before peeing in his pants. Friday, he was lucky—he held it in, but he had to run from the bus to the bathroom. He made it there, just in time.

Finally, a good morning: Nathan's test results were blue, which is normal. He was excited, and he got to sleep in because it was Saturday. He went downstairs, and his mom was already up, making breakfast. He turned on the TV to watch the morning cartoons. Nathan's dad came down a few minutes later, and they ate breakfast together as a family. Breakfast was good, but he didn't remember what they had. He did, however, remember going over to Neil's house and meeting his mother, who was very nice. She offered Nathan a drink, which was some sort of fruit drink. Nathan knew that he wasn't supposed to have sugar, but he didn't want to make a scene. He also didn't care as much, so he drank the punch. He recalls how good it was and how, in the moment, it was worth the risk of going to the bathroom several times.

Neil showed Nathan his room, and it was full of toys. He had a really cool Matchbox® (toy cars, not the ones you start fires with) collection and toy soldiers. They took them outside to play. Things then became uncomfortable for Nathan. He had to pee again. "Not now," he said to himself. He decided to hold it in because he was having such a good time. He didn't want to screw up his friendship because of his diabetes. He lasted for another half hour, until he felt it more strongly than before. He then asked Neil if they could go inside and asked where the bathroom was. Most of the urine ended up in the toilet. The rest didn't show through his pants. Nathan decided that he wouldn't tell anyone as he worked hard to hide his diabetes. He told himself, "I will be normal again."

While still in the bathroom of his friend's house, he dried his underwear using the toilet paper in the bathroom, and he didn't mention it to anyone. He spent another hour or so playing with Neil in his room. Neil's mom called up and asked whether they wanted brownies. They both ran downstairs and picked from the plate of brownies his mother placed on the table for them. They were the best brownies Nathan had ever had. He couldn't wait to get asked back to Neil's so he could get some more of them next time. They watched a little TV in Neil's living room until it was almost time for dinner. Nathan unfortunately had to go home, and he had to pee again. He really had to work on holding it in. He confessed that he did go back for seconds on the brownies. He said that they were so good. Anyway, he thought, besides the urinating issue, he did great and had a great day. Nathan had thought to himself, "I hope I will be able to control my urination better next time."

MONDAY, SEPTEMBER 1, 1980

Well, it's a new school year. For Nathan, last year was tough to get through. He must have peed his pants at least fifty times during the school year, most of which was in the first three months. He worked very hard to control his bladder. He thought about how long he could hold his urination, for at least two hours, and that it must be a world record, but he couldn't tell anyone. Nathan created a routine around the bathroom and his classes that by the end of the year worked pretty well. He was a little nervous about it, but he was sure he would make it work. "Have to. No one knows, and I intend to keep it that way."

SATURDAY, SEPTEMBER 27, 1980

Nathan had been out of control since his grandfather passed away a week earlier. For the past week, he had been riding his bike to the candy store and binge eating. He hadn't urinated this much since he first got diabetes. Nathan realized that no one noticed.

SATURDAY, OCTOBER 18, 1980

A few days ago, Nathan's dad left on a business trip. Before leaving, he showed Nathan how to draw up his own shot. While his dad was away, Nathan discovered that he could still eat lots of candy, and if he increased his dosage, he wouldn't be as sick. After his dad's return, Nathan's father was so impressed at what a good job he had done, he told him that from now on he could draw his own shots and give them to himself. Nathan's mom was supposed watch him test his urine, but she only asked what his test result was. Of course, Nathan would lie and say that it was great or close to great. Nathan believed at this moment of his life that he had made the greatest discovery on the planet: how Nathan, a child with diabetes, could cheat and get away with it.

CHILD'S PERSPECTIVE

Going back to school with the diabetes diagnosis was scary for Nathan. He feared that his friends would not want to play with him and that he would have been left all alone. He was scared that he would spend the rest of his life by himself. Nathan felt isolated and distant from his classmates, as though they had already abandoned him. He felt overwhelmed with fear and worried about what would happen if he failed to take care of his diabetes. He felt that his parents hadn't noticed his pain. This belief was unknowingly reinforced by his mother, a month after leaving the hospital, when she said, "You are doing so great! You are being so responsible about taking care of your diabetes."

Every day throughout his childhood, Nathan wished that the responsibilities of living with diabetes were taken away from him. He stated in a session with me, "I was just a child! I was pretending to be brave. I was scared, petrified, and felt all alone, so alone." For Nathan, and any child, peeing his pants is humiliating, to say the least. He was mortified.

During that session, he continued to talk about his fears. He felt they were insurmountable: "The doctors all told me that high blood sugars could kill me. The excessive urinating was a constant reminder that I could die." He said that he felt all alone with his problems. Worst of all, he no longer felt like a child.

His parents would also fight a lot. In response, he would have feelings that he was the cause, along with his diabetes, because he was a burden to them. Feelings like the world was on his shoulders led him down a destructive path, which led to eating lots of candy to feel happy, if only for a few minutes.

Due to Nathan's out-of-control diabetes and the negative emotions that were not addressed, he felt hopeless and tired all the time. Feeling very alone in the world with an illness no one he knew could understand, he spent a lot of his childhood wishing he would wake up one day and it all would have been just a bad dream.

PARENTAL ADVICE

In the beginning, when getting home from the hospital and in the days and weeks that follow, parents should be vigilant about asking their child how he or she is feeling and let the child know you are there for him or her. To raise a healthy child, diabetes care needs to be a team approach.

Children need to feel that they can talk about their feelings and that it is normal for them to have these, whatever they may be. Regardless of the feeling or the problem that is causing it, they need to know that they are not alone and that you will work with them to resolve the issues that happen together. They need to know you will listen to them and that they are heard, in a nonjudgmental environment.

Remember, nothing with diabetes runs smoothly, especially in the beginning. If your eight-year-old child is behaving like an adult when managing his or her diabetes, you may have a problem. Conversely, if your child is not listening to you at all and is eating candy daily, then you may have a different problem. You are doing okay if your child is doing what you ask of them, for the most part, even if every now and then he strays from his diet or forgets to give himself insulin. A common example is when they have cake without giving insulin to cover the additional sugar intake because their friend brought in cupcakes for the whole class and they wanted to fit in.

You are the adult, and you need to help your child manage not just the physical aspects of diabetes but also the emotions and how to handle situations that come with it. If you are struggling with helping your child, or your child is struggling with emotional issues beyond your ability to help, it is okay to seek help. You can also seek help if any family member, including you, is struggling with emotional issues related to your child's diagnosis.

"Flexibility Is the Key to Your Family's Happiness"

If you don't want to be angry all the time, it is important to remember that your child is just that—a child—and will behave like one. You will face many issues with your child with diabetes. It is important to not be reactive to the situation or your child. He or she didn't ask for it and shouldn't be punished for behaving like a child in light of it. Neither should you. Regardless of what happens, keep your cool and remember that your child may not understand the consequences of his or her actions. Children need to feel that they are understood, listened to, accepted, and feel like a normal child for their age.

Adapting to your child's needs may become crucial to your family's happiness when raising a child with diabetes. Support your child by making it okay for him or her to ask for help at home, at school, and anywhere they happen to be. Encourage them to ask for help from others. For Nathan, all he had to do was tell the bus driver that he needed to go to the bathroom, but since he didn't feel that he could open up to his parents about it, how could he open up to anyone else? Instead, he suffered needlessly.

Since high blood sugars are a common problem for children growing up with diabetes, it is important to tell your child that it is okay to ask to go to the bathroom. As a parent, actively follow up with the different systems that your child will be interacting with so each of them can support him or her in what may otherwise be an uncomfortable situation. For Nathan, it may have been the school and bus driver. Every child with diabetes will have high and low blood sugars, but how we react to that news as parents plays a big role in whether your child will feel safe enough to be honest about what is happening with their blood sugars and other issues. Blood sugar levels are neither good nor bad; rather, they are markers (data) to know what course of action will need to happen next. High blood sugar with no "insulin on board" (how much insulin that is still active in your child) requires a correction bolus, whereas a fasting blood sugar of 50 may require, depending on other mitigating factors, fifteen grams of carbohydrates. If you use the terms "in range" and "out of range" as information to help your child, determine what they need to do to get back in range and inform the child instead of chastising him or her for not being in range; then your child is more likely to come to you when his or her blood sugar is not in range to seek your support. Attaching the label of "bad" to a number implies to that child with diabetes that he or she is bad. Since no child wants to get in trouble, they are more likely to keep the high and low numbers to themselves in order to avoid causing any issues with their parents.

With Nathan's situation, he said that his bus driver was really nice, that he felt comfortable talking with him, and that he probably could have spoken with him about finding a way to work together so that Nathan could have gone to the bathroom when he needed to. Basically, you don't know if you don't ask. No one in this world is going to come and ask you whether you are okay, so teaching your kids to be advocates for themselves is very important. It is just as important that their parents, like you, be advocates for them too.

CLINICAL ADVICE

Communication is the key to all successful relationships. For children with diabetes, open and nonjudgmental communication is critical to your child's safety and success.

Communications Skills (Vary Dependent on Age)

1. Always start with "I feel . . ."
2. Keep your statements short—no longer than one minute—and focused on one point of the issue at a time.
3. Respond by rephrasing (paraphrasing) back to your partner or child what they said and ask whether you got what they said right. If accurate, then you respond to the feeling statement. If inaccurate, then ask for the feeling statement to be restated.
4. If accurate, respond only to the statement made and for no longer than one minute. Stay on the topic presented. Respond with concern and empathy. We are dealing with your family's feelings. The goal is for everyone to feel listened to and appreciated.
5. Then have your family member or child rephrase what you said, and ask whether they understand what you said. If they don't, try to rephrase your statement.
6. Repeat until you have addressed the issue, come to a compromise, or have a plan of action. (A lot of things may need to be discussed, but don't put all of it in one conversation, as it can be overwhelming. Address only one issue at a time.)

Example: older child (twelve to fifteen years old):

a. I feel sad when I see other kids eating candy and I am not allowed to have any.

b. So you're upset that your friends get to eat candy and you don't. (Rephrasing) Is that it?

c. Yes, I don't know why I can't have what they have.

d. First, let's talk about why you are sad and then we can address the issue of eating candy. (Staying on track)

e. Why do you feel sad when you see the other kids? (Exploring the feeling)

f. I feel alone and left out! Why did I have to get this horrible illness?

g. So you feel you are alone with this problem, and when other kids get candy, it puts it in your face. (Staying on track and rephrasing: you can always return to a new topic—this horrible illness—that comes up in the conversation after a solution to the present topic has been reached)

h. Yes, it makes me feel alone.

i. Was there something specific that made you feel this way? (Exploring what triggered the feeling)

j. In school, there was a birthday party before lunch, and everyone got cupcakes. (The trigger)

k. You must have felt very alone. (Showing empathy) How about you and I come up with a solution so you don't feel left out next time? (Join with your child)

l. Sounds good. I really wanted to eat a cupcake with the other kids.

m. Did you know that there was going to be a party ahead of time? If you did, we could have adjusted your meal plan ahead of time. (Exploring the issue and possible solution)

n. No, I didn't know.

o. What if you ate a cupcake with the kids and then bolus (pump) insulin to cover or give an extra injection to cover the extra carbs? (Plan of action)

p. Sounds great!

q. If you do that, it may also help if you reduced your carbs at lunch. (Plan of action)

r. I can do that!

s. Great! If you still feel sad or left out, I am here for you. (Keeping lines of communications open)

t. Thanks, Mom.

u. You're welcome. I will always be here to help you out if and when you need to work through a problem. (Reinforcement)

v. So you also brought up that you didn't understand why you have this horrible illness. Do you want to talk about that or should we save that for another day? (Not everything needs to be solved now and shouldn't be)

Example: younger child (eight to eleven years old)

a. Why are you crying?

b. Some kids made fun of me.

c. Where is this happening? (Clarification)

d. In class.

e. Are the kids in your class teasing you? (Rephrasing and confirmation)

f. Yes.

g. Do you know the reason why these kids were making fun of you? (Exploration)

h. No.

i. What happened in class before you were teased? (Exploration)

j. Johnny's mother brought cupcakes to class. Stupid teacher!

k. Why are you angry with your teacher? (Exploring the feeling, address language later in conversation)

l. She was handing out the cupcakes. When she got to me, she said I couldn't have any because I have diabetes, right in front of everyone!

m. Did the other kids made fun of you because you were not allowed to have a cupcake? (Summarizing the event and confirmation)

n. Yes.

o. You must have felt alone and left out! I am sorry this happened to you. Let's see if we can prevent it from happening again. (Showing empathy)

p. Stupid diabetes!

q. Yes, it is a bad illness, and it is horrible that you have it. (Paraphrasing with empathy) How about you and I come up with a solution so you don't get left out next time? (Redirecting back to the topic at hand and joining with your child)

r. How?

s. I can talk to your teacher and the school nurse to explain that you can have cupcakes and other sweet foods as long as right before or right afterward you go to the nurse and have her adjust your insulin. (Plan of action)

t. Okay. What if it happens again?

u. I am pretty sure this will work, but if not, we will figure it out together. Okay? (Joining while keeping the lines of communications open)

v. Okay.

w. *Hugging your child*

x. Now, how about we go out and get you a cupcake for a snack?

y. Chocolate?!

z. Yes, a chocolate cupcake.

aa. Yay!!!

bb. Before we go, it's important that you don't call your teacher or anyone else names. Do you think you can do that?

cc. I can do that.

dd. Great! Let's get you that chocolate cupcake!

ee. Thanks, Mom.

ff. You're welcome. Your father and I will always be here to help you out when you need us. (Reinforcement of team approach)

gg. *Save tips for how to deal with a bully or talking about your child's feelings about having diabetes for another day.* (Not everything needs to be solved now and shouldn't be)

Deescalating the Defiant Child

TUESDAY, FEBRUARY 12, 1980

It was a special day for Charlie; it was his ninth birthday. He didn't know when he started cheating on his diet, but it was about a year ago, around his eighth birthday. In late summer or early fall, his father took Charlie aside and said that his parents were getting a divorce. He thought it must have been sometime in mid-October, based on when the divorce papers were signed. Charlie's dad said, "I will be getting an apartment near the house, and we will get to see each other on weekends. It will be great. You'll see. Great!" He told Charlie that Charlie would be staying with his mom. He said that he loved Charlie and that it had nothing to do with him, but Charlie knew better.

THE VICTIM

He knew that they were lying. It had everything to do with Charlie. His father was leaving, and it was his fault. Maybe if he had done something different, then his dad wouldn't be leaving. Charlie thought that if his parents didn't need to spend all their time dealing with his diabetes, then his father wouldn't be abandoning him. He wasn't upset about his parents getting a divorce. He was more terrified of being left alone with his mom. Charlie's mom was very strict, while Dad was the fun parent; he definitely wanted to go with his dad.

In retrospect, wanting to go with his dad had nothing to do with who his mother or his dad was, but rather his attachment to his dad. Charlie's dad did a lot with him, like teaching Charlie to ride a bike, play tennis, shoot toy rockets into the sky, and more. He spent a lot of time with Charlie until he left the house when Charlie was eight years old.

He wasn't there because of the divorce; it had nothing to do with Charlie or his diabetes. It took Charlie a long time to realize this because memory is a tricky thing for a child with diabetes. It was difficult for Charlie because his high, low, and shifting blood sugar levels interfered with his ability to think clearly and remember. When blood sugar is high or too low, a child will have a hard time retaining or remembering new information until the blood sugar returns to normal. It happened all the time to Charlie.

His dad's departure caused him to feel abandoned, which inevitably led Charlie to cheating on his diet and a process addiction. After Charlie's father told him that he was leaving, he felt sad and angry. A little later, that anger turned to rage. "I'll show them. I'll make myself so sick that they will have to stay together," he said to himself. He remembers that day as if it happened yesterday. Charlie left without saying goodbye and started riding his bike from Tulip Grove Road, down Harkness Lane, and then turned up Center Way Road. Somewhere between Center Way and Montgomery Village Avenue, he started crying and continued crying until he arrived at his destination: Walkers Choice Road. It was uncommonly cold for the time of year, without a cloud in the sky. He got off his bike and threw it to the ground. Then Charlie walked into a store that would be his secret for the next five years, where he would pick up his drug of choice: lemon drop candy. He looked on the rack and saw a bag of the lemon drop candy and bought it with his allowance. Charlie felt good walking out of the store. He knew that his parents didn't know about the convenience store, and he felt in control of his life. The chaos that was surrounding Charlie started to drift away. The rush of it all was exciting. He sat on the curb and started to eat the candy. Charlie got concerned that his bike was out in the open for everyone to see. He took his bike and moved it around to the back of the store. He found a sturdy tree near his bike and sat down, leaning against the tree. He reopened the bag of candy and proceeded to put another lemon drop in his mouth and bit down. Eating the candy felt euphoric to Charlie! As he crushed his teeth into each piece, he felt better and better until he forgot the reason for eating the candy in the first place.

He didn't come close to eating the whole bag, so Charlie took the rest home. The round trip was about three to four miles from his house. From then on, he made that trip at least once a month and spent his entire allowance on candy. He didn't always buy the lemon drop candy, although that was the cheapest. During the months when Charlie had more money because he had stolen it out of his mom's purse, he would buy chocolate and other types of treats too. This time was the first of many that Charlie would steal either money or (later on) cigarettes out of his mom's purse.

LOCUS OF CONTROL (ONE'S PERCEPTION OF INNER AND EXTERNAL CONTROL)

On the ride home, Charlie felt empowered and in control. When he got home, his mother was angry and started yelling at him. He didn't care. She wanted to know where he went, and he told her, "I walked to the creek at the end of Harkness Lane, then up to the pond where I cried. Then I came back home." She calmed down and said that she was just worried about him. He asked whether he could go up to his room, and she said that he could. As Charlie went up to the top of the stairwell and then turned the corner, he felt euphoric. He had gotten away with it all and was proud.

DANGER OF ADDICTION

In a session, Charlie stated with glee, "I had gotten away with it, and it was the first of many lies. It just rolled off my tongue! So easy!" The truth is, he hadn't gotten away with it after all. Before dinner that day,

Charlie's mother handed him a test strip, and he went into the bathroom. He tested his urine, as blood testing for the general public wasn't available yet. The strip turned dark brown. Dark brown meant high levels of sugar were in the urine. If his blood sugar was normal, the test strip would have turned light blue, but it changed from blue to green to brown. He then read the chart on the bottle of test strips to see how high it was. It was so brown that it was even darker than the chart indicator.

His mother asked him how he was doing. With his head hung low and guilt written all over his face, he left the bathroom to face the music. His mother saw the test strip and was angry. With teeth clenched, she slowly asked him why the strip was so dark and what he had eaten that could have caused it. Charlie said he didn't know why his blood sugar was so high (lie 2). She asked him to tell her what he ate that day. He told her everything, except the candy (lie 3). Charlie couldn't recall much after that point, but he said he made a pact with himself to never let that happen again. He would test his blood sugar level before his mother had the chance to ask him to do it and tell her what the results were—or at least his version of them.

At one point, his dad found out. Charlie's father felt that if he had approached him about his cheating, he would have cheated even more. He didn't want to push Charlie away or risk losing his relationship with his son. As he recalled everything that was going on during that time, Charlie could understand why. However, his dad might have been the only one Charlie would have listened to. If his father was able to articulate how dangerous it was, using just the right words, Charlie might have stopped cheating.

MASTERMIND

As time went by, Charlie started getting better at cheating. One of his favorite lies was the fake low blood sugar reaction. Having low blood sugar meant he needed sugar or he would end up in the hospital unless he could raise it—and what better way to get candy or ice cream than faking a low blood sugar reaction? It worked like a charm.

When his blood sugar was too high, Charlie would say he must have eaten too much. He played with the gray zone. Most of the time he would give extra insulin at dinner to cover up the blood sugars. After his dad left, and since his mother didn't play much of a role in his insulin injection, Charlie was in total control of that part of his life. He could eat as much candy as he wanted and get away with it.

HALLOWEEN PAST, PRESENT, AND FUTURE

According to Charlie, "Halloween night was great!" He got tons of candy. Since he could no longer have it every day, he was looking forward to it more than ever. It started like every other Halloween. He was excited with gluttonous anticipation.

The day before, the other children at school were talking about previous hauls. He didn't realize that he was going to have to give his candy to his mother. Charlie remembers crying inside as he handed the candy over to his mother. His mother reminded Charlie that they had agreed that they were going to exchange toys for candy that year. Charlie's mother thought the toy idea was great; Charlie wished he had felt the same way. When it came down to handing in the candy, he didn't want to. The toys were not as important to Charlie as fitting in at school.

He couldn't understand why this had to happen to him. At that moment, he hated having diabetes. Charlie pictured his friends and schoolmates unwrapping their bounty and enjoying every moment.

He was right. The next day at school, everyone was talking about the wonderful candy they got, comparing how much of it they collected, and who got the best kinds. Charlie was very quiet at lunch because he only got toys and had to give up his bounty of candy. That Halloween was not so great, but things would soon change.

After his dad left, Charlie got away with a lot more. Charlie's mother was working hard, and he was helping out around the house, even getting dinner ready for when his mother would get home. He was seen as a good kid and very responsible for his age. When he was ten years old,

Charlie was staying home alone after school. As the next Halloween approached, he knew one thing—this year would be different.

He was going to fit in again. He told himself that, but it was only an excuse, a lie to justify what he was about to do. By that point, he had been lying and cheating for over a year and lied about anything and everything. It was compulsive, but so convincing that his lies were never proven. He quickly became very good; it was pathological in nature. In truth, he did all of this for the candy itself. He loved it more than anything or anyone, and at that point it was his only source of happiness.

UNDER THE BUSHES

On Halloween day, before Charlie's mother got home, he placed a bag under and behind the shrubs in the front yard. This year he went trick or treating with his next-door neighbor's kids. He went dressed as Dracula, and he had a lot of fun. "What a haul, so much candy of every kind," he said to himself. He waved goodbye to his neighbors and watched as they entered their house. Once the coast was clear, with a wicked grin he walked to where he had left that bag earlier that day. The candy he didn't want to eat stayed in the bag his mother bought for him to use. He put a few good pieces in the same bag since he felt that she would never believe that all he got was raisins and candy corn. After leaving his secret bag hidden under the bushes, Charlie went inside his house, and his mom asked him how he made out. "Not as good as last year, but it doesn't matter. What toys did you get me?" he asked with excitement in his voice. Charlie didn't remember which toys he got. He did remember wanting to go back outside so he could bring the secret bag full of candy into his room so he could start eating it. He was overly excited. While tempted, he knew that if he wanted to pull this off, he was going to have to wait and stick to the plan.

THE PLAN

Charlie went to school the next day and said what he got. When a teacher overheard his conversation, he told her the truth, as he always did—just not the whole truth. Once the teacher and Charlie were out of earshot of the other kids, he said, "I did get all that candy," to the teacher, who had a frown on her face. Then she asked, "Does your mother know you have all that candy?" "Yes," Charlie said. "I handed the bag to her, and I got one piece and a toy. Then she threw the rest of the candy away. Please don't tell the other kids. They will make fun of me. Please don't tell." Charlie started to cry, and tears were streaming down his cheeks. "Of course, I won't!" she said as she handed Charlie a piece of candy and said, "One little piece won't hurt." (Did I mention yet that Charlie had learned how to turn on the water works at any time? It came in handy many times during his childhood.) The rest of the day at school went okay. All the children were staring at the clock, counting the minutes until they could go home to their candy.

Charlie got on the bus, sat in his usual spot, and had an uneventful trip home. After the bus dropped him off, Charlie looked around to make sure that the coast was clear. As planned, he was the first one home, and the neighborhood was deserted. He walked toward the hiding spot, and the bag was still there. He grabbed it, brought it inside, and placed most of the candy in his hiding spots around the house. Some went into the air vents, as they had central air conditioning. The next hiding spot was in his bed under the mattress between the wooden slats, and his last spot was in one of his Humpty Dumpty toys. He didn't say how exactly he did that one—just know that Charlie was as good at hiding his candy or maybe even better than an alcoholic who hides their booze. He took a few pieces out to eat right away, and the rest went into hiding. A week later, it was all gone. As time went on, the schemes got more complex, and so did the lies.

CHILD'S PERSPECTIVE

Charlie blamed both of his parents for not protecting him. He was angry with them, diabetes, and himself. "Why can't I be like the other children? It's unfair!" Charlie would say this to himself at his friends' birthday parties, when the ice cream truck was on his block, and at any other event where he was not able to eat what the other children were having. Living with diabetes made Charlie feel isolated and different from the other children. Throughout his childhood, he struggled with feelings of isolation. He just wanted to fit in.

According to Charlie, his mom recalls that he used to avoid playing with the other children after being diagnosed with diabetes. His mother also remembered how she didn't worry much about him because he acted more mature than the other children his age.

While Charlie was growing up, he felt that everyone, even strangers, could see that he had diabetes. It was as if he had a big sign on his back that said, "I'm a child with diabetes. Feel free to pity me!" Charlie spent a lot of time in his room after getting diagnosed with diabetes, feeling sad and alone. After making sure that his parents were downstairs, he would lie on his bed and cry. He felt dead inside and refused to accept his diabetes diagnosis. While on the outside Charlie always tried to show that he was totally accepting of his diabetes, which worked out great for his parents and those around him, it caused him great pain and sadness inside. "I'm fine! No need to worry about me! No need to pity me, because I am fine and I can take care of myself."

The first time Charlie was allowed to have candy after getting diagnosed with diabetes, he was elated. It felt so good that he wanted more right then and there, but he wasn't allowed. That is when the anger started. It felt like the whole world was against him. By that point, Charlie felt that candy equaled happiness. So on that fateful day during October 1980, he kicked his cheating into overdrive. At first, the cheating made Charlie feel good. When he would start to cry, he would take out a piece of candy and eat it, and then the pain would go away for a while. After some time had passed—he couldn't remember how long after the first time—the candy no longer helped his pain, anger, sadness, fear, and self-pity. During this time in his life, everything was crazy and out of control for him. As an adult, he knows the reason why he kept doing it: even after he knew that the repercussions of cheating were more painful than the pain the candy resolved in the first place, it was the only thing that Charlie felt he had control over.

Charlie tried to be everything to everyone else: the perfect child, son, student, and so on. When he was twelve years old, his mother realized that he was depressed. Charlie, who had been diagnosed with diabetes three years earlier, finally got help to manage the issues his diabetes had created for him.

PARENTAL ADVICE

Charlie's mother never found out about the cheating until Charlie told her when he was thirty-six. His mother was surprised to find this out. His dad, however, knew about it but felt that if he had approached Charlie, it would create conflict and cause Charlie to push him further away from him, leading to even more cheating. Both his mother's denial and his father's fear of abandonment caused Charlie to feel that his parents didn't care that he was alone with his diabetes. So the question is: What is the best way to address cheating?

Punishment won't work because your child is covering his or her feelings up with candy, so further stress and anger will only drive them further toward the candy. Punishment includes talking down to your child; yelling, cursing, hitting, or spanking them; or taking away anything the child values. Luckily, a combination of various techniques will help reduce your child's cheating.

Addressing the Addiction

First, do not use the term *cheating* while addressing the issue or refer to his/her behavior as wrong or bad. It is normal for a child to want to be like all the other children and eat candy and other sweets. Have an open discussion with your child about why they are "eating candy," which may involve how they are feeling about having diabetes. Discuss what eating candy and other sugary snacks does for them. The more understanding and sympathetic you are toward their reasons for "eating candy," the easier it is to address and, chances are, the more they will be willing to talk with you about it.

Remember, a punishment doesn't address the cause and just creates more reasons to cheat. Talking about your child's feelings with him/her, how he/she is coping or adjusting to his/her diabetes, and the reasons he/she has turned to binging on sweets will yield better results. The goal here is to make your child feel supported and loved.

You need to foster a delicate balance between independence and making all the decisions for your child. Children need to feel that they have some level of control. While discussing these issues, express that you are there for them and that they can approach you even if you seem busy. If you are busy, you can always tell them that you need to finish up what you are doing and will find them when you are done. It is important to compromise, within reason, with your children around the management of their diabetes.

Openly discuss their feelings with them. Listen to them. Show your child that he/she is not alone and that you will help him/her solve the problems together. The greater communication you have with your child, while helping him/her find healthy coping skills, the less likely it is that he/she will turn to eating sweets when feeling angry, sad, or out of place. With better coping skills and the knowledge that he/she can come to you when problems arise, the more likely it is that your child will come to talk with you before turning toward candy. When they are hurting, even adults will turn to what makes them feel good (i.e., ice cream), even if they know it is bad for them. Eating sweet things for a child with diabetes is an unhealthy coping mechanism for negative feelings.

Balance is the key to happiness in life. This is also true when managing diabetes. Better balance in all aspects of life will cause fewer high blood sugar episodes, less shifting of blood sugars (stability), and fewer low blood sugar incidents. Better diabetes management equals fewer mood swings and a higher chance that diabetes won't affect proper brain development. It also reduces disabilities, increases your child's IQ, and improves his/her ability to focus, giving your child the same chance to succeed as kids without diabetes.

It is important to discuss how to handle blood sugar, insulin, and food management with your child. For a younger child, who may not have the ability to manage as much, it is important to help them with various diabetes management tasks so they can maintain a good physical and emotional balance. With older children who can take on more responsibility, they may need emotional support but may not need help with the management of the physical aspects of diabetes.

Internal fighting among family members is not helpful, especially when it centers on your child's diabetes. Each family has to find its own balance. Not everyone is going to be happy with the house rules, but always keep in mind that you are the parent and that you need to make choices that are best for all of your children. For example, healthy food is good for everyone, so avoid making it about the diabetes.

Charlie would fight with his mother about weighing food. The more they would fight, the angrier he would get, and the more he would binge on sweets. Instead of finding a compromise, his mom wanted Charlie to weigh his food and match the quantity of food to how much insulin he took. He wanted a more adaptive style of management, allowing him to eat as much as he felt like and then match how much insulin to give based on the quantity of food he ate. Letting your kid live a normal, comfortable life that meets his/her needs doesn't mean that he/she can overeat and do whatever he/she wants. You are still the parents. If age appropriate, allow your child to base his/her insulin off an adaptive style of management. Remember, this is about compromise and trust. My best advice when integrating diabetes into your household is to adapt diabetes needs into the existing house rules that your children already follow. An example is to slowly change the diet of the whole family. Abrupt change may cause other household members to blame the child living with diabetes. Don't make special rules for diabetes; instead, adapt diabetes requirements into existing rules. If you already allow your child to have McDonald's once a week, continue that rule. Change the insulin to match the carbohydrates for that meal. A child with diabetes should not eat sweets on a daily basis, but no one really should. Give them a choice for the type of treat they can have and agree on the quantity of sweets they can eat weekly, thereby making them part of the decision-making process. Give them a feeling of control. Your child will be more invested in taking care of their diabetes and less likely to cheat. For example, if you are going to McDonald's and your child living with diabetes wants to eat an apple pie but their friend's birthday party is tomorrow, give them a choice of whether they want to eat an apple pie now or save their treat for the birthday party tomorrow. You are not changing the rules; you are simply adapting to life changes.

CLINICAL ADVICE
Cheating on diabetes and how it relates to addiction is addressed below.

Addiction
The main entry for *addiction* in Merriam-Webster is as follows:

1. the quality or state of being addicted
2. compulsive need for and use of a habit-forming substance (such as heroin, nicotine, or alcohol) characterized by tolerance and by well-defined physiological symptoms upon withdrawal; broadly: *persistent compulsive use of a substance known by the user to be harmful* (http://www.webster.com/dictionary/Addiction)

Addiction is a dependence on a behavior or substance. Addiction in the past has focused mainly on alcohol and drug dependency. More recently, researchers have started to recognize other addictions. There are two classifications of addiction: chemical dependency, which usually includes alcohol, illicit and prescription drugs, nicotine, and certain over-the-counter medications; and process addictions, which can be sex, gambling, shopping, and eating disorders such as bulimia or anorexia.

The substance itself doesn't create the high; it is the chemical change that occurs in the brain, causing an increase of dopamine. Dopamine occurs naturally in the body to reduce stress and anxiety. It is our body's "Joy Juice." This "Joy Juice" releases naturally without drugs. The body naturally produces dopamine every time a person eats or exercises and during any activity that causes an individual to feel good or elated. Unfortunately, drugs artificially cause the body to produce dopamine at a much higher level than can be produced by the body naturally. When we compare sex to methamphetamines, the stimulant drug causes the brain to release over five times more dopamine than sex. After a while, tolerance to the drug builds up in the body, and the body becomes programmed to release dopamine only when that drug enters the body. Tolerance is one of reasons why most people who are living with addiction no longer enjoy sex, food, or exercise during early recovery.

In my time spent in the field of addiction as a psychotherapist, I have had several people with diabetes as patients who used drugs to compensate for the negative feelings of high blood sugar levels, which cause depression and a severe lack of motivation. Usually cocaine, marijuana, or alcohol is used to self-medicate. But where did the behavior start? It is different for each person. Charlie never used cocaine to self-medicate, but he did use nicotine in his teens to his early twenties. He presently has two decades of sobriety under his belt. Charlie did have one slip since he quit twenty years ago: He bummed a cigarette off another New Yorker who was also looking down Park Avenue in New York City, watching the smoke, fire, and ashes rise out of the ground on September 11, 2001. However, he stayed strong and didn't revert to his process addiction, binging on candy.

One addiction can lead to other addictions. Charlie's binge eating had started to subside but was replaced by cigarettes. In session one day, he said, "Thank God no one had introduced me to cocaine. It would have been the end of me."

The Process of Addiction

Process addictions are addictive or repetitive behaviors that interfere with several aspects of life. Process addiction still creates a chemical reaction, releasing dopamine. Like substance abuse, it is self-medicating, and one of the only real differences is the mind-altering effect that comes with most drugs.

Some children with diabetes are addicted to sugar and cheat on their diet daily and, for example, will eat a box of Ho Hos or Twinkies in one sitting or binge on a bag of candy. Unlike gambling or an internet addiction, it is both a process and a chemical addiction, with sugar as a mind-altering component. In people living with diabetes, the severity of binge eating is huge. High blood sugars cause the brain to slow down due to less oxygen reaching it. Less oxygen causes reality to drift away. So, in English, your mind is in a fog and can become a hiding place where your child's feelings go when they are upset.

Binge eating is a dysfunctional pattern of eating caused by emotions, which consists of episodes of uncontrollable eating. During a binge, the person eating rapidly consumes an excessive amount of food. A bulimic will compensate for the effects of overeating by purging. Purging is enacted through induced vomiting or laxatives to undo the previous behavior. There is a process that is similar to bulimia when children who are living with diabetes cheat. The child with diabetes either eats high-sugar food or binges without thinking about the consequences and then, after the fact, compensates for that behavior by giving more insulin.

There is a type of binge eating that doesn't fit into the addiction category for people living with diabetes. The "diabetic binge" I am referring to occurs due to chemicals that get released by the body when blood sugar goes low. The chemical normally releases when the stomach is empty and causes the sensation of hunger. Unfortunately, low blood sugar also causes the body to produce this chemical. The chemical doesn't shut it off until the blood sugar returns to normal, and it can take twenty to thirty minutes after the chemical shuts off for the hunger to subside. The lower the blood sugar level, the more intense the feeling of hunger. This, along with the cognitive impairment caused by low blood sugar that impairs judgment, can lead to binge eating—the perfect storm.

If low blood sugars are not involved, binge eating may be part of a process addiction. For someone with diabetes, it becomes a way to cover up his or her emotions. It is very different from having a planned treat once a week, when insulin is given ahead of time to control for the treat. Cheating involves impulsivity, and insulin is injected after eating. Sometimes the person will allow their blood sugar to rise to a very high level. Once they feel sick, they give a shot, and not the correct amount, as it is harder to get extreme blood sugars to come down. The normal insulin sensitivity ratio doesn't work well at this time. The process hurts their health and continues to produce negative consequences in every area of their life. Therefore, cheating (binge eating) becomes a process addiction.

My definition of process addiction is an obsession with a behavior utilized to fill an emotional void or suppress or cover emotional pain. It is spontaneous but done in a rigid manner for immediate satisfaction and relief from emotional pain. For someone living with diabetes, it interferes with physical and emotional stability, causing excessive amounts of emotional pain. Eventually, the child starts lying to cover and conceal, maintaining the behavior for instant gratification. Lying to oneself and others when signs of the problem become transparent is the result of the process.

Process addiction for binge eating has four components:

1. Emotional or physical pain
2. Absolute thinking about relieving pain: "Only binging will alleviate my pain!"
3. The binging causes a short-term reduction of pain
4. The binging causes a long-term increase of pain

Charlie's Addiction as It Relates to the Four Criteria

1. His emotional pain regarding his diabetes along with the unavailability of his mother and his parents' divorce fit the first criterion. He was feeling guilty because he thought his diabetes caused their divorce. Diabetes led to feelings of loneliness, which caused him to isolate from other children. This was a lot of pain for a young child, and his father's abandonment triggered his usage. He was angry and was going to show them.
2. After more than a year of having these feelings, Charlie had finally found that the only way to relieve his pain was through the candy he ate that fateful day in the early fall of 1980.
3. Candy fixed everything for Charlie. It cleared the tears from his eyes and made him happy. He was no longer focused on his feelings, but rather on the next hit of candy and the candy he was eating at that moment. He spent countless hours avoiding his feelings of anger and isolation through figuring out where and when he was going to get his next score and constructing elaborate plans.
4. Charlie reduced his immediate pain, but in the end it was all consuming and hurtful. The cheating itself caused several problems physically, cognitively, emotionally, and socially in both the short term and the long term.

If your child is already cheating/binge eating, it is important to recognize that doing so is addictive. Seeking help for your child from a specialist such as a licensed clinical social worker who is certified in alcoholism and substance abuse may be a good place to start. Check with your endocrinologist or general practitioner for a referral.

Navigating the Impact of Out-of-Control Blood Sugars

During our third session, Sandy said, "Okay, so I have told so many lies as a child, even I couldn't and still have a hard time recognizing what is real and keeping all the lies straight." What Sandy had said so far was the truth as she saw it as a child and as an adult. So, where to start about the complications Sandy faced on a daily basis until she stopped lying and cheating?

THURSDAY, NOVEMBER 1, 1979

Let's start with the day after her third Halloween since that horrible day in the hospital when she received her diagnosis: diabetes. Sandy knew that her bag of candy was waiting for her at home and was excited. Before this, her blood sugars had been high a lot because of her cheating. One of the symptoms of the onset of diabetes is dehydration if untreated. On any given day, Sandy would have to urinate on the hour every hour, thanks to all the sugary snacks she ate. Some days were better than others, but that was an average. This leads up to the bed and bus/van incidents. To the best of her recollection, Sandy was around eight years old the day after her third Halloween with diabetes.

NO HARM, NO FOUL
The bus ride home the day after Halloween was exciting but worrisome
to her, but that day by late afternoon, things were not looking so good.
Sandy started thinking, "What if my mom found out? What if she is waiting to catch me in the act? What would my dad think of me?" Sandy felt
so guilty, and she hadn't even eaten one bite of the candy she'd hidden.
After getting home that day, Sandy found the bag right where she had
left it and took it inside to her room. She dumped the bag of candy on
her bed and ate several pieces right away. Then Sandy realized the time
and felt it would be awful if she were caught. Sandy then left her room
with the bag of candy in tow and started hiding it around the house, going from one hiding place to another: from the garage to the basement
to the attic to the heating vents. Then she thought, "What if Mom turns
on the heat, the candy melts, and the chocolate smell goes through the
house?" Sandy was freaking out—big time. In the summer, the heating
vents were the best place to hide candy. There were just two screws to
remove, and the vent came off. It became a storage unit for her: put
candy in and screw in the two screws—done. In a panic, Sandy decided
to eat the candy (binge) before Mom got home. "So good, so good," she
thought to herself. Sandy was in heaven. She had half an hour to eat
everything. She was back in her room, sitting on her bed, focused on
nothing but eating it. Sandy was only halfway through the candy when
she suddenly heard her mom's car pull up. Sandy ran out of her room,
and back in, then left again, and then got halfway to the steps when she
realized "THE CANDY!" It was on the bed. She ran back into her room
and hid the rest of the candy, plus the loose wrappers. Her mother came
home in her usual bad mood after work. Sandy realized that her mom
was too wrapped up in her own problems to notice what she had been
up to. Yes, she got away with it, and so no harm, no foul.

THE CALM (FEAR) BEFORE THE STORM
As the minutes until dinner ticked away, Sandy watched television and
kept a close eye on her mom. Paranoia started to set in as the clock told

her it was a few minutes until dinnertime. Dinner went on as normal, making her even more paranoid, as if her mother had read her mind and was waiting for her to get comfortable before striking. Sandy was worried all night. It was one of the longest nights of her life. In her mind, the perfect plan was falling apart. By the end of dinner, Sandy was apprehensive and asked whether she could play in her room. Her mom said yes. Sandy thought to herself, "Did I? Did I get away with it?" Sandy cracked a smirk on her way up the steps that night. She was so happy that after all that worry, her mom didn't know about the candy. The hiding and sneaking were over, but in about a half hour, the real hiding would begin.

THE STORM

During the night, the complications of high blood sugar levels set in. Sandy had known about these complications since the day after she snuck off to the candy store located near her house and binge ate about a pound of assorted candy. Sweets made her feel so good that Sandy didn't care about the consequences of binge eating candy. Sandy went to the bathroom a lot that night. It was hard to remember a number or how many times she went per hour because her mind was clouded and spinning. She felt sick to her stomach. The only way to describe the feeling was that she felt hollow inside. Her body was weak, and Sandy couldn't stop drinking water.

Sandy was hiding from her mom in her room. As Sandy expected when she started feeling sick, a half hour later she found herself sneaking off to the toilet to urinate and drinking lots of water from the bathroom sink. Her mom was downstairs in the living room watching the evening news. She hoped that her mother wouldn't notice her little problem. Sandy didn't flush when using the toilet because of the noise. Before leaving the bathroom, she would turn on the cold water and drink from the faucet for up to five minutes or more. In Sandy's mind, it felt like she was in the bathroom for hours at a time.

Eventually, her mother yelled from downstairs that it was time for bed, and Sandy needed to brush her teeth. She would be up in a minute to say good night. Sandy went to the bathroom and brushed her teeth. She urinated again, this time flushing the toilet, and then changed into her pajamas and got into bed. Her mother said good night as she normally did, and then she went back down to finish watching television, not suspecting anything unusual.

At that point, Sandy realized that her mother didn't know and that she was sick for nothing. Sandy was furious with her mother and her diabetes for causing her to hide her candy in the first place. She continued to pee often that night and listened very carefully for her mom, who came up an hour later to get ready to go to bed. Sandy sat by her door for what seemed like hours, waiting and listening for her mother to get into bed and go to sleep. Several times her mother would come close to her door, and Sandy would run back into her bed. Eventually, Sandy saw the light from under her mother's bedroom door go off. Sandy went to the bathroom again; she peed slowly, making sure that her peeing wouldn't be heard. Before sneaking downstairs when she was done, she drank more water, and then she tiptoed down the steps and headed toward the kitchen. Sandy thought, "It's time to fix this problem," and then . . . she tripped over her cat, Mittens. His cry was so sharp and loud; Sandy thought she was done for. She lay still, not making a noise for five minutes. When she heard no footsteps coming down the stairs to yell at her for not being in bed, she thought, "Maybe it's a trap," but nothing. Her mind was still spinning as Sandy went into the closet and got a syringe. Then she went into the refrigerator to get regular insulin and kept it open for light. By the refrigerator light at midnight, she drew back the plunger on the syringe, watched the precious, life-saving insulin draw in, and then pulled the needle out of the bottle. Giving the syringe a flick to remove the bubbles, Sandy paused and said that she would never do this again. (Lies, lies, and more lies.) Sandy pulled the string that held her pajama pants up, and they instantly fell to the kitchen floor. With her pajama pants around her ankles, Sandy pinched the injection site on her leg, jabbed the syringe into her leg, and pushed the plunger down. She felt the cold rush of the insulin entering her muscle and quietly let out a sigh of relief. Even today, Sandy still likes the feeling of the cold insulin as it enters her body. However, Sandy was worried that she would take too much; she was new at drawing and giving herself injections. If she were to have a low blood sugar reaction while sleeping, she worried that she might go very low and wake up in the hospital. Sandy wasn't concerned about her health; she just didn't want to get caught. If she had known how many calories she had eaten, Sandy might have given more, but she didn't. Based on the next twenty-four hours, she should have. Once back in bed, Sandy fell asleep fast.

FRIDAY, NOVEMBER 2, 1979: THE STORM RAGES ON

At five in the morning, Sandy woke up in a pool of urine! Every now and then, Sandy would pee the bed (high blood sugars suck), but this was one of the worst times. It wasn't because she couldn't get up and go to the bathroom. It was a choice. When your sugar is high, you have to get up every half hour to pee. If it goes on too long, you may give up, say "screw it," and let it happen. On some nights, like this one, Sandy would wake up, decide not to stop urinating in bed, and go back to sleep.

On this night, though, Sandy had had several dreams about peeing, but she only remembered one clearly enough to tell about it: Sandy was swimming in the ocean. It was summertime, and a riptide was taking her out to sea. She looked to the shore and saw her mother yelling something over and over. Sandy eventually heard what she was saying: "That's what cheaters get." She was struggling to get back to shore and found it too hard. Sandy let go and eased into her fate of drifting out to sea, and it felt surprisingly good. A few minutes later, she started to cry. Sandy realized in her dream that she was lost at sea, and the waves were getting rough. Sandy woke up in horror, crying, and in a sea of her own urine. After a few minutes, she calmed down and understood that she had urinated in her sleep—and had done it more than once.

NO ONE TO HELP HER AFTER THIS HURRICANE EITHER

Once Sandy got up, she knew what to do. She took some dirty towels from the laundry hamper and threw them on the bed. She waited as they soaked up the urine. Sandy then used another towel to wrap the linens and took them down to the basement. She put them in the washing machine, threw in some detergent, and pressed "start." Sandy heard the machine roar to life and headed upstairs. On the way back to her room, she stopped by the closet to pick out some fresh linens, grabbing two pillowcases and a new set of bed sheets. She then made her way back to her room. Her mother was still asleep as she passed her room. Sandy quietly made the bed in her room and then headed toward the bathroom to pee again. She came back and decided to put a towel down on her bed, just in case she couldn't make it through the last hour she had left to sleep before she had to get up. When she woke up, the bed was still dry. Sandy thanked God. (For those of you who are wondering about the wet mattress, stop wondering. Remember, this was not Sandy's first diabetes-related incident involving peeing in the bed, so her parents had put the plastic mattress and plastic-covered pillows on her bed long ago. The plastic made the bed so much easier to clean up.)

THE AFTERMATH

Sandy went downstairs and ate breakfast. Her mom avoided cooking at all costs, so it was no surprise that it was plain Cheerios cereal with saccharin. (Um, can't you just taste the cancer? At the time, it was what was available as a sweetener for those with diabetes, and who knew?) Sandy went to the bathroom right after breakfast. She was about to walk out the door when she realized the time and bolted out instead. Sandy got to the bus stop just in time to see the bus drive away. She was worried what her mother would say, but instead of yelling, her mom simply said, "No problem, I'll drive you to school." Soon they were on the way to her elementary school in Rockport, Maine. Sandy and her mom usually didn't talk much during the ride, which would have been a good thing today, but on this morning her mom wouldn't stop talking to her. Her mom's need to chat was a problem during this trip and became very apparent the moment Sandy noticed the pressure on her bladder. It is very hard to focus on not peeing for half an hour and speaking at the same time. "Warning, kids, don't try this at home."

When they arrived, Sandy kissed her mother goodbye and ran into the school, right into the bathroom, ignoring some teachers who said good morning. Such relief came over Sandy as she urinated. It was a good time to go, before class, because the only way to make it through the day without questions was to pee between class periods, which she took advantage of during all seven breaks.

Sandy's challenge was insurmountable; she sat through several classes with her legs crossed, wishing the bell would ring. Sandy normally daydreamed in most classes. She always paid attention in math for at least the first half of class, but today was especially hard. Math was something she was good at, so it wasn't surprising for her to be called on by the teacher to go to the front of the room to solve a problem. However, today of all days, with only five minutes left, she was called on to solve a problem on the chalkboard. Normally, she would be glad to go up to the board and write the answers; instead, this time Sandy asked whether she had to. The teacher said that she noticed that Sandy wasn't paying attention and wasn't raising her hand to answer questions during her lessons. Sandy begged her again to let someone else respond to the question and that tomorrow she would be happy to answer extra questions. Just then, another kid in the class said that he would go up. The bell rang before the teacher could get another word out. Before the teacher looked back at her, Sandy was up and out the door on her way to the bathroom. Sandy felt bad, but she didn't care; the bathroom and toilet were all she wanted.

Sandy proceeded to her next class and was looking forward to recess. She was walking up to the baseball field to play kickball during recess—her favorite game. Then, all of a sudden, Sandy felt wet and realized she had started to pee her pants. "I can't believe I am nine years old and still peeing my pants," Sandy thought to herself. She felt humiliated and told herself, "I am useless and stupid." Sandy squeezed her bladder hard, stopped urinating, and ran to the bathroom, crying as she peed in the toilet. Luckily, it wasn't much, and only her underwear was wet. Lucky thing, because no one liked her at school to begin with, and the last thing she needed was for the other children to tease her. While crying, Sandy thought, "You are so stupid! How could you forget to go to the bathroom first? You are so worthless. This is why you will never amount to anything!!!" She would say this over and over.

Sandy was hiding these episodes. For every time that her parents found out there had been one, there were at least nine more incidents they didn't know about. It was how she learned to sort whites from colors in the laundry, especially reds, when washing clothes.

After spending a half hour in the bathroom yelling at herself, she headed back to play kickball. Everyone was heading back and laughing at what a fun time they had. Dread set over her. Sandy had already said it all in the bathroom. After she heard her classmates laughing, she felt so sad and alone. Sandy started to cry and held the tears back. On the way back to class, she felt ashamed and stopped by the bathroom again. Was this going to be her life?

HER REALITY

All the kids knew about her peeing problem (they really didn't; Sandy just felt that way), and a few kids did tease her on the playground from time to time, more often than she cared for. She spent a lot of days on the playground alone. Leaving the playground and school behind that day wasn't difficult. Sandy went to the bathroom and had to be the first on the bus. It was always the same bus: a white van with green lettering that read "Rockport Country Day School."

Every day she would sit in the same spot: in the second to last row, the furthest seat in, for one and only one reason. Was it the best seat? No. The kids next to her were typically dropped off first, and she knew that she would be the only one who would be sitting there peeing her pants. It was embarrassing enough on its own, but having someone else sit in her pee would be devastating.

On this day, Sandy made extra sure that she was on the bus first. Typically, if Sandy peed herself, she could stop it. Stopping partway did two things: she got some relief to make it home, and only her underwear would get wet, so no one would know. Today was no ordinary day, as you can see. There were others, but none quite like this day. Literally two minutes before reaching home, Sandy peed her pants so bad that she left a puddle. Her embarrassment was huge, but since she was the last stop, Sandy just got up and left the van.

Unless Sandy missed the bus, she had to ride it both ways. She was the first one picked up and the last one dropped off. Unfortunately for Sandy, it was an hour-long bus ride each way.

Sandy walked home. She had a couple of hours before her mom got home, so she washed her clothes and took another shot of insulin. Sandy went up to her room, laid on her bed, and cried. It was over, and she was crying. That made her feel worse, and she started saying how weak and sick she was. Sandy felt like everyone knew and everyone was going to point when she went back to school. She didn't know what her blood sugar was because they only had test strips for urine when Sandy was a child. Her guess would be in the 500s ml/dg. She started feeling better physically around the time her mother got home. No one ever called her mom to say what had happened during her bus ride home or during school. Sandy was relieved.

SOME LIGHT THROUGH THE CLOUDS

The math teacher looked at her in a funny way the following Monday, as Sandy would raise her hand to answer every question. The odd thing was that Sandy got called into the principal's office after math class. She thought it was for the incident that had happened last week in math. They had all her tests in front of them and went through them one by one. Her grades were 102 percent out of 100 with extra credit, 105 percent out of 100 with extra credit, and 100 percent with no extra credit given. Sandy looked at them as if they were crazy; she hadn't done anything wrong. Hers were the best grades in the class. All of a sudden, as if they knew what she was thinking, the principal said that he had heard from most of her teachers that she spent her class time looking out the window and daydreaming. Sandy got scared that they were reading her mind. She thought they knew what had happened with her blood sugars. Fortunately, the school was unaware of her blood sugar issues. Her situation at school was worse, however, than if they knew. They said that she needed to pay more attention in class, but it appeared that she had a gift for math. They opened her math book and saw that she was more than halfway through the book, and it was only November 5. The principal said, "Maybe they aren't challenging you enough?" Sandy said, "You are! No! You are challenging me plenty!" (not realizing that his question was rhetorical). He ignored her shouts and response. He said that she needed to have more focus in all her classes. Sandy recalled the principal giving her permission to no longer pay attention in math class, but she would have to continue to work at the same or an increased pace in the workbook and text. After finishing each chapter, she was to tell the teacher, and she would give Sandy the test. Sandy loved math. It was the only other subject besides art that she enjoyed. So, Sandy agreed, but the principal said, "While we are here, let's talk about your other classes," like English and social studies.

F OR C, IT IS ALL THE SAME, LOL

By December, Sandy still hadn't gotten her grades up in English and so-cial studies, but this was a private school. Even if you failed, you passed with a "C." It happened in first, second, and third grade. It would and did happen again, so who cared? However, because of what had hap-pened that day in class, her high blood sugars helped her get her math talents noticed. As a result, by December 14, she had completed the textbook for the year, and she felt good for the first time since getting diagnosed with diabetes. Sandy was then given the book for fifth-grade math. The following year, she skipped a grade in math class and was put in sixth-grade math. But as Sandy entered fifth grade, her mother was becoming increasingly upset with her work and quit her teaching job. Her mother then took another job in a different state. When they moved, Sandy was forced to change schools.

At her new school, they tested her academic competence in all subjects. She scored at a sixth-grade level in math, but her reading and writing skills were at a second-grade level. Her poor grades were a direct result of the cognitive impact of continuous high blood sugars. The inordinate amount of time and energy she spent dealing with her out-of-control blood sugars also affected her grades.

A BRIGHT SPOT

If it weren't for her worst high blood sugar ever that consequently impacted her ability to focus in math class and caused her teacher to think she was not challenged enough, Sandy would not have experienced the self-confidence-building moment of getting acknowledged for excelling at math by her school, which helped her feel that she could succeed in life despite her diabetes.

CHILD'S PERSPECTIVE

Cheating: Sandy felt that she had no choices. She wanted to be like her peers, but she wasn't old enough to express her feelings of isolation. Sandy was paranoid about getting caught. She lied so much that she had two lives: the real, sad one and the good little girl. Guilt, oh, the guilt Sandy felt, so guilty that she thought she was the worst daughter ever. Sandy was angry. She felt punished for having diabetes. She started to isolate herself and watched "caretakers" do it for her. The bullies on the playground made her feel helpless. The caretakers she talked about included her parents (who limited what she could do), school officials and teachers (who told her what she could or couldn't do in front of her peers), and her doctors.

She felt that she had less control over her life than all her peers. All children want to feel some level of control over their life. She didn't think or care about the physical and emotional impact of cheating. She knew about the health risks, but, like most young children, she didn't understand them or the meaning of death. Sandy felt indestructible, as she was able to lie and get away with it so often. She believed that she was invincible until her late teens. The longer Sandy lied and cheated, the lower her self-esteem became, but succeeding at lying gave her a false sense of being able to do anything and a false sense of control.

Peeing in bed and in her pants caused continued feelings of isolation and separation from her peers as well as profound sadness. High blood sugar led to frequent urinating, and it took away so much of her self-esteem. However, Sandy learned that she could temporarily relieve the pain through eating yummy treats to avoid her sadness.

Succeeding in math: This was important because her diabetes (and most people's) causes biochemical damage as well as physical, emotional, social, and self-esteem damage. In her case, Sandy's self-esteem was a big problem, but being good in math was great. Sandy felt good and worked harder at math until she was doing sixth-grade math in fifth grade. Sandy was on top of the world! Math gave her hope.

PARENTAL ADVICE

My best advice is to stop it before it starts, when possible. What rules around food and snacks existed before diabetes? Ideally, nothing should change when your child with diabetes comes home from the hospital. If you allowed McDonald's one time a week and three treats weekly, continue this routine and adjust the insulin to match the lifestyle your child is used to. Do not change it abruptly. If you have McDonald's daily, that is bad for anyone, and your family would benefit from seeing a dietitian/nutritionist. Change everyone's diet in the family slowly, and avoid having a different diet for your child living with diabetes.

If you believe that your child is already sneaking sweets and living with the consequences that Sandy went through, it is important to remain calm. Anger never helps. You will be fighting an uphill battle. If handled properly, you can win the battle with much less of a fight. Every child is different, so your approach needs to be adjusted accordingly.

In Sandy's case, I would recommend addressing how she was feeling about having diabetes. Did she feel responsible for it or punished by it? I would let her tell you her feelings and then validate her feelings: "If I had to live with diabetes, I would feel that way too." Be supportive by saying, "I want to help and we will figure it out together. You are not alone. We are in it together. Regardless of what happens, you can talk to me, even if you think you will get in trouble. I promise to listen to what is happening and not get angry at you because this is all new for me too." What you say may look like this or something like this or nothing like this, but what is important is being congruent. Your behavior needs to match what you tell your child. If you say you are going to be there for her, then you need to put the time in and be there, without judgment.

Remember, diabetes management requires adult decision-making skills. Therefore, children will make many poor choices as they are learning how to manage their diabetes, friends, and the world around them. As a parent, you are not there to punish, but rather to help correct and teach your child how to make better choices.

If you are struggling with what to say, revisit the advice given in chapter 4 of this book about communication. It is important to have an open dialogue with your child about how he/she feels. Once your child knows you are going to be there for her, which may take time, she will start coming to you about the problems she faces, and it is important to help her realize that the world is her oyster, and how she has the same opportunities and options as the other kids, and that having diabetes doesn't have to make her different from her classmates.

Have a weekly family meeting to discuss how everyone is feeling in general and around any household changes or new rules, as well as talking about the positive things you and your children can look forward to. In these meetings, avoid talking about diabetes, unless your child brings it up. While your other children need to know some aspects of the diabetes, they don't need to (and shouldn't) be involved in every aspect. The end goal is about normalizing diabetes and helping your kids fit in with their peers. Continual communication is crucial. If you don't know how or have poor communication with your children or another family member, seek out a family counselor/psychotherapist.

CLINICAL ADVICE

We are going to look at the short-term complications of type I diabetes and the immediate consequences of high and low blood sugar.

Hyperglycemia (hy·per·gly·ce·mi·a) is an abnormally high level of sugar in the blood. The immediate cognitive consequences are a lack of focus, lack of concentration, depression, poor attention, daydreaming, below average grades, poor memory recall and retention, lethargic behavior, and slow thought processes. Physical consequences include increased levels of thirst, dry mouth, hunger, increased urination, weight loss, weakness, fatigue, blurred vision, skin that is dry or itchy, frequent infections or cuts, and bruises that take a long time to heal.

Your child's blood sugar level can climb for numerous reasons. This includes eating too much, being sick, or not taking a sufficient amount of insulin. To avoid hyperglycemia, check blood sugar levels often and watch for the above signs and symptoms.

Most common symptoms include:

Increased thirst and frequent urination: As excess sugar builds up in the bloodstream, fluid is pulled from one's tissues, which may leave your child thirsty. As an effect of this process, your child may drink and urinate more than normal.

Extreme hunger: Lacking adequate insulin to move sugar into the fat cells causes the muscles and organs to become depleted of energy. This depletion triggers intense hunger that can persist even after eating, because without insulin, the sugar never reaches the body's tissues, like our muscles.

Weight loss: Despite all the eating, the muscle tissues use up all the fat stores for energy until they are depleted. The body then looks for another source for energy, using tissue from the muscles themselves for energy, causing the muscles to atrophy as well as an unhealthy loss of weight from decreased muscle mass.

Fatigue: When cells are deprived of sugar, a child with diabetes many become tired and irritable.

Blurred vision: When blood sugar levels are too high, fluid will be extracted from all tissues in the individual's diabetes body, including the lenses of one's eyes. This affects the ability to focus clearly (MayoClinic.com).

Diabetic ketoacidosis: When one's cells are starved for energy, the body may break down fat, producing toxic acids (ketones). As stated above, this will cause loss of appetite, nausea, vomiting, fever, stomach pain, and a sweet, fruity smell on the breath. To prevent ketoacidosis, check your child's urine for excess ketones. There are over-the-counter ketones test kits to check for these. If your child has high levels of ketones in their urine, reduce their blood sugar levels using insulin. Due to various factors that happen during ketoacidosis, more insulin than normal (about 50 percent more) will be needed to correct for the high blood sugar levels. Your child should also be drinking eight ounces of water every thirty minutes. No-sugar/carb sport drinks or vitamin water that are high in potassium are also good to reduce potassium loss while restoring and prevent hydration. If high levels of ketones continue for more than four hours or your child is vomiting, call your child's endocrinologist right away and then go directly to the hospital.

If your child has continuous hyperglycemia, you may need to change their meal plan, insulin regimen, or both. If they are consistently above 250 mg/dL regardless of changes, seek advice from an endocrinologist right away. There is a condition that causes this situation called hyperosmolar syndrome, a life-threatening condition in which very high blood glucose levels cause the blood to thicken.

Hypoglycemia (hy·po·gly·ce·mi·a) is the medical condition of having an abnormally low level of sugar in the blood. If left untreated, low blood sugars can cause seizures, loss of consciousness (coma), and (on rare occasions) death. The immediate consequences are weakness, sweating, shakiness, hunger, dizziness and nausea, drowsiness, slurred speech, and confusion.

When one's blood sugar level falls below the target range, it is recognized as low blood sugar. It can reduce for many reasons, including missing a meal or snack, above-normal physical activity, or taking too much insulin. Even short walks will burn carbohydrates and cause blood sugars to decrease, making it important to adjust carb intake prior to the walk or during the walk with a snack and always have glucose on hand while monitoring blood glucose levels closely. It can also occur if one takes insulin too soon before the Chinese delivery guy arrives with the food that was ordered. Check your child's blood sugar often, and watch for initial signs and symptoms of low blood sugar. Early signs are muscle weakness, shakiness, dizziness, sweating, hunger, and nausea. Later symptoms consist of slurred speech, drowsiness, and confusion. Hypoglycemia at night causes sweat-soaked pajamas or a headache because of sweating. If night sweats are occurring on a regular basis, test at 2:00 a.m. to confirm the blood level and call your child's endocrinologist.

When your child has symptoms of low blood sugar, make sure they eat or drink things that will swiftly increase their blood sugar level, such as glucose gel, tablets, or powder, as well as hard candy or another simple carbohydrate. If your child loses consciousness, you may need to give them an emergency injection of glucagon, which is a hormone that stimulates the discharge of sugar into the blood. If you are not familiar with this treatment, consult your child's endocrinologist for more information and instruction.

7

Managing Low Blood Sugars

I turned forty-seven years old today and realized that I have lived with diabetes for forty-one years. Over that time, I, too, have had many experiences living with diabetes. Like my client Mary from chapter 2, I received my diagnosis on my birthday. It was an interesting moment in therapy when Mary disclosed that she was also diagnosed on her birthday. As I reflect over the past forty-one years, I thought it would be helpful if I included some memorable moments of my life with diabetes as well.

SUMMER OF 1980

This summer was when I had my first experience with severe hypoglycemia unconsciousness/coma. I remember little about the experience except that it was one of the scariest moments in my short eight years of life. What I do remember is that it was uncomfortable, to say the least.

It was a warm, sunny afternoon, and I felt exhausted. I remember lying on my bed and falling asleep. I was awakened a short time later by my mother, who was shaking me, and her boyfriend, Tom, who was standing behind her. Tom was a six-foot, eight-inch black man who was my favorite of her boyfriends. He was a gentle giant. He rolled me on my side while my mother ran and got the shot of glucagon (liquid sugar). While Tom was holding me, my mom pulled my pants down and gave me the shot in my butt. I remember Tom kept telling me over and over again that everything would be all right while he stroked my hair. It was comforting to hear, but I didn't believe him. I passed out again and then woke up in Tom's arms as he carried me through the kitchen and out of the house to my mother's car.

What I remembered next was waking up in the hospital and feeling like crap. My first memory of that hospital room was seeing my mom and her asking whether I was all right. Without responding, I leaned over the side of the bed to find an ideally placed bedpan. A split second later, I proceeded to throw up into that bedpan. Afterward, everything faded out again. From time to time, I would wake up and lean over the side of the bed to find an empty bedpan, which I gladly filled up again and again throughout the night. As the evening progressed, I fell back to sleep for longer lengths of time. I was relieved when morning came and the vomiting ceased.

THE DAY AFTER

The following morning, I felt very nauseous, but at least I had stopped throwing up. It felt like I had the Ebola virus. My mother took me home, and a day later, I felt better. Before leaving the hospital, I was told by the doctor that it could have been much worse and that I was to watch my sugar levels more carefully. If I felt weak, he told me to check my urine often. I knew one thing: I would definitely be checking my sugar levels. I never wanted to go through that again.

EARLY SPRING OF 1983

Three years after my first trip to the emergency room, I found myself surrounded by giant mice and ducks. I was so excited that my mom and I were in Disney World for vacation. I had been waiting for this trip for months. We finally arrived in Florida after countless hours of me begging her to take me during the past year. It was early afternoon when we walked out of the airport in Florida. The drive to the hotel went quickly. I even saw a place called Wet and Wild on the way. Wet and Wild was the largest waterpark in Florida, with a one-thousand-story-tall water-slide that was so tall I almost hurt my neck looking at it. My mother said that if I was good, we could go there before heading back home.

THE RIDE

After checking in, we unpacked and decided that there wasn't enough time for a visit to Magic Kingdom (the original Disney World), but we could go over to Epcot. I remember walking under the monorail with my mother as we entered Epcot. It had only one or two rides at the time, and the rest of it was very boring, like the foreign pavilion. My mom was excited by the displays, but I just wanted to go back to the hotel. After I had complained incessantly (in my head and maybe once or twice out loud) about how bored I was and what a stupid place it was, my mother turned to me and said that there was a great ride we hadn't gotten to yet. I kept walking and followed her to a ride that had a one-and-a-half-hour wait. I never got to go on the ride because it was late, I needed to eat, and I unfortunately realized that I had left my shot in the hotel room. At this point, we decided to call it a day.

I was angry about forgetting my shot, which caused me to complain even more about how stupid Epcot was and how it had no real rides at all. With a look of disgust on her face, my mother said, "Well, we're not going back! Let's just get back to the hotel room." I was happy to get out of there. (Full disclosure: I have had many friends who went and loved Epcot at various points during their lives. I never went back.)

I remember walking under the monorail on our way out, wishing we had taken it to Magic Kingdom instead. At the time, I was probably a little too young to grasp Epcot. After getting back to the hotel, I watched TV, my mom read her book, and then both of us were off to bed. I did another urine test before bed. It was abnormally high for me, so I gave a little extra insulin in my shot, and then I crawled into bed and fell fast asleep dreaming of the awesome rollercoasters I would get to ride. I still love rollercoasters—the faster, the better.

EVERYTHING IS UNDER . . .

[*Back in the 1980s, doctors cautioned that being higher is better than having a low blood sugar reaction. Today, higher is not necessarily better. As a young adult during my college years, I realized that the higher blood sugars caused many problems, both emotionally and physically, that led to unnecessary grief. During my childhood, I barely realized the impact of high blood sugars, except that they tended to make me urinate a lot along with feeling tired and sad.*]

On day 2 of the trip, I woke up, tested my urine, and saw that my blood sugar was high. I didn't realize at the time that sugar from a previous high could remain in your bladder until your next urination, and I hadn't urinated all night. I added extra insulin to my breakfast bolus to cover the high blood sugar I most likely didn't have. It was a sunny day out. We went down and ate breakfast in the hotel restaurant. After breakfast, we returned to our room, where my mother was taking forever to get ready. I was frustrated but also excited because in about an hour, I was going to be at Disney World. Twenty minutes later, I was tired and dizzy. My mom had me check my urine just before I started feeling ill. While the urine strip showed the lowest results it could possibly have been, I didn't say anything. I don't know what I was thinking, and I guess that is the problem when you are out of control. I just kept lying down on the bed and falling asleep, but my mother kept trying to wake me up. Someone gave me a glucagon shot somewhere between my mom calling 911 and arriving at the hospital. It was all a blur.

Next thing I remember, I was waking up in the emergency room. My first memory of this emergency room was not seeing my mother and thinking she had left me. I thought to myself, "She went to Disney World without me." Then I started throwing up like the last time into yet another bedpan. Then everything faded out. I would wake up every now and then to vomit and then fall right back to sleep. My mother was eventually allowed to see me. Shortly after that, they discharged me.

[*In my first six years of dealing with diabetes prior to blood testing, I had learned how to prevent prolonged periods of high blood sugars by testing my urine and giving shots to adjust. I am not sure that attempting that was the cause of my trip to the hospital in Florida. After this experience, I realized that there were dangers in playing catch up with insulin that peaked four hours later.*]

TYPHOON LAGOON

The day after, I was still feeling woozy and nauseous, and Mom felt we needed a rest. She followed the doctor's advice and decided that we should take it easy that day, and that is what we did. It was a fun day at a water park. No, it wasn't Wet and Wild, but thanks for the positive thoughts.

Disney's Typhoon Lagoon Water Park in Walt Disney World Resort is where my mother chose to lie in a chair, sunning herself all day, and I got to go down various rafting rides. I have to admit that I wasn't happy when my mom suggested it, but it was a lot of fun. I ultimately was glad we went there. I was feeling much better at the end of that day and looked forward to going to Disney World—at last—tomorrow.

WE MADE IT!

The following morning at the hotel room, I felt fine, but my mother still asked whether I was ready for Disney World. Well, you probably know what my answer was. We went on all the rides, including some kickass rollercoasters. That day I was extra careful about my diabetes. Around noon, my legs started to feel weak. I told my mom and didn't try to hide it from her. When I checked it, my urine test showed that my blood sugar was low, so I asked whether I could get some cotton candy. My mom said okay. By 3:00 p.m., I was feeling down and a wave of nausea was coming on. I checked my blood sugar again, and I was high. I gave myself a shot of insulin, but it took the rest of the day for me to recover. I was even looking forward to the Huckleberry Finn boat ride by the end. It was a beautiful, slow-moving ride.

On the fourth day in Florida, I finally got it right. That morning I planned a little better. I cut back on my NPH insulin, which is my longer-acting insulin, in anticipation of all the walking around. I was finally feeling better, and I started to enjoy Disney World. By the last day, my blood sugar levels stabilized in time for the plane ride home. Don't tell me that that didn't suck, but, all sarcasm aside, it was a learning experience. I still managed to have a great time.

EARLY FALL OF 1993

It was my last year of college at Frostburg State University, located in Frostburg, Maryland. I was sharing a duplex with my best friend, Larry, and his girlfriend, who was a real b***h (mean person). This was my first duplex house. It was crazy, like someone built a house, cut it down the middle, and then put a giant wall up. We lived in the right half of the house, and three guys from Baltimore, Maryland, lived on the left side of the house. One of the neighbors became a good friend of mine, and we had some good conversations while sitting on the porch.

As you walked into our place, the separating wall was on the left. On the first floor, the bathroom, living room, and dining room were on the right side, along with stairs that led to the bedrooms upstairs. There were two large bedrooms with lots of space. Mine was on the right as you went up the stairs, with a western view, and Larry's bedroom was on the left.

While the bedrooms were huge, the living room was tiny. You had to go downstairs to use the bathroom. The kitchen/dining room had an island with stools to sit on. At the end of the long hallway that ran along the dividing wall, there was a back door that led from the kitchen to a big backyard where we grilled once in a while. To me, the duplex was fascinating, because if you entered our next-door neighbors' apartment, it was a mirror image of our apartment with everything to the left.

I was twenty-one years old at the time, and I was finishing up a bachelor's degree in fine art with a dual focus on painting and design (my first career). Everything was going as planned. My best friend and his girlfriend (who, as a reminder, was mean to me during that time) and I were living in that duplex right off campus. The three of us would share the chores, including cooking dinner, but for breakfast and lunch everyone was on their own. On this particular night, it was Larry and his girlfriend's night to cook, and I was studying for a big test I had to take the following day.

It was about mid-October. While studying, I started daydreaming about school ending and enjoying the summer off before heading to New York to become a successful artist. Because of my attention deficit disorder (which had been diagnosed nine years later) or diabetes, or a combination of the two, I would have to read each paragraph two to three times before I could remember the material. I think I was studying a chapter for my sociology class.

FROM NORMAL TO STEPHEN KING

I had been studying all morning, and it was now about 3:00 p.m. I was still unsure whether I would pass my upcoming midterm. I was having more trouble than normal reading at my desk because of the two windows that surrounded it. The one in front of the desk faced the front of the house (a western view) and the one to the left looked out the right side of the house (a southern view); both had warm sunlight coming through them. All I could think of was "Wouldn't it be nice to be outside today?"

I started to feel tired and laid down on my queen-size mattress that I had bought at Goodwill for $20. There were no other parts of my bed, not even a box spring. I had placed the mattress on the floor to the right as you walked in the room. It was along the wall that faced the stairs. It was not the most comfortable—a little lumpy and hard to get out of—but that day it felt like heaven. I had been studying all day and just assumed that that was the reason I was so tired. I lay down and fell asleep. About an hour later, I woke up.

I was very groggy and went downstairs. I asked whether anyone had seen my toothbrush and said that I was going to bed for the night. Not waiting for a response, I went upstairs, fell back onto my bed, and started to shiver. Every muscle in my body began to feel shaky. Larry came into my room two minutes later and asked whether I need help. I said, "Did you find my toothbrush?" Larry tried to get me up, but he couldn't and I didn't want to. I just wanted to fall asleep so the shakiness would go away.

The next thing I didn't know, in that moment, was that I had become paranoid and delusional and was hallucinating. The paramedics came into my room, and I thought they were minions of the devil coming to hurt me for not studying. I pushed two of them across the room as they tried to get me out of my bed. A few seconds later, three cops came into my room. At the time, they didn't look like cops to me, just more minions coming to get me. One of the cops tried to restrain me, and I pushed him across the room as well. Then Larry came back in and said that they were here to help. I called him a traitor and asked how he could turn me in.

While distracted by Larry, the two other police officers and the other paramedics grabbed me and strapped me to a plank of wood. (Later I realized it was a gurney.) As they carried me down the narrow steps, I noticed that the walls were on fire. I felt the heat from the fire, and I was coughing from the smoke. No one seemed to notice or care.

As we got to the bottom of the stairwell, I tilted my head back to look at the fire. All I saw was an empty staircase. I was shaking violently. One of the paramedics lost hold, and I fell. During the few seconds that I was lying on the floor, still strapped in but on my side, I saw flames start to shoot up the wall that divided the two apartments. I screamed, "Doesn't anyone see the fire?!" and no one responded.

I was still lying on the floor in the entranceway to my apartment. I started to say to Larry, "Aren't you going to . . . ?" and then the fire went out. The wall was black and parts of the wall looked like melted wax on the side of a candle. Still coughing from the smoke and lying on the ground, the wall started to change from my perspective, and the room began to shake. Various faces started to protrude out of the wall. The bulging faces started talking to me, saying things like "You're going to hell, young man!" and "It's all your fault! You are going to die, and no one can save you now!" I screamed, scared beyond belief, but nothing came out—just silence.

The demons picked me up. I was still strapped to the board as they proceeded to take me out the front door. Looking back at the house, I heard a demonic voice come from the interior of the house saying, "No one can help you. They can't hear you in hell."

Many people were looking and laughing at me as they took me to a hearse. One onlooker said, "You're going to die!" When we got to the hearse, I realized that it was Larry who was holding the door to the vehicle. As they slid me into the back, he said, "It was nice knowing you," and then slammed the door shut. I thought death was coming and blacked out.

UP THROUGH THE RABBIT HOLE

I awoke in a room no bigger than five feet by eight feet. The cinderblock walls were cold to the touch and painted white, very intuitional. Still strapped to a gurney, I couldn't move my arms or legs. I felt like I was Jack Nicholson in the film *One Flew Over the Cuckoo's Nest*. Sometime later some orderlies came into my room to take off the straps and slid me into a hospital bed. A few minutes later, a nurse came in, and I told her that I felt weak. I asked whether I could have some orange juice. The nurse said no and then picked up a giant syringe and stuck it into my arm. Laughing a little, she said, "Pure glucose will do the trick." I screamed and thrashed about as the intense pain went shooting up my arm.

I started shouting for my friend Larry, saying that if they didn't get Larry, I would rip the IVs out and find him myself. I then started screaming, "Larry!!!! Where are you??!! Larry!!!! Larry!!!! Larry!!!! Where are you, Larry?! Larry!!!!" Then, finally, Larry walked in (sporting a black eye) with a different nurse. I started to calm down. Larry walked over to me and gave me a hug. As he hugged me, I felt safe again. I wanted to go home. I asked the nurse whether we could go. She checked my blood sugar levels and left the room. Larry helped me to sit up, and I thanked him for being there. I asked him what happened to his eye, and he told me that I punched him when he tried to give me some orange juice. I apologized, and he told me not to worry about it.

We talked for an hour about how scared I was and what I thought was happening. He said that when I had asked whether he and his girl-friend had seen my toothbrush, I was actually holding it. I stood there for at least two minutes, just staring at them. I had then gone back upstairs. I hit one of the paramedics, so they got some cops to come in to help. I was then focused on the cops. I pushed them back, and the paramedics used that distraction to get me on the stretcher. They saved my life. I never saw them again, and if somehow this gets back to you, thank you. Larry said that I seemed out of it. He had tried to help me, but after I had punched him, he called 911. A doctor came in to the hospital room and said that I was good to go but warned me that I should watch my blood sugars carefully over the next week. Larry took me home. My arm was all bruised from the shot, and if this somehow gets back to that nurse, I hope that you found compassion for others over time. This was my last episode of a diabetic seizure, but not my last experience with diabetic seizures.

Fast forward, and I was now living in New York City, trying to make it as an artist. My friend Judy had juvenile diabetes and was not in control of it. She was sick a lot, and from time to time I would ask her when she last checked her blood sugar levels. Most of the time I would get the same answer: "No, but I feel fine." I knew she wasn't. I could see the changes in her behavior and attitude, as people had seen it in mine when my blood sugar was high or low.

One night, Judy was to meet me and my girlfriend (at the time) and my best friend Holly at a great burger joint in New York City. The four of us had plans for dinner at 6:30 p.m. and then we had tickets to see an off-Broadway play. Judy didn't arrive for dinner, and it was now about 7:00 p.m. The show began at 8:00 p.m. Holly and I were about to go looking for Judy when a strange man came into the restaurant and asked for me. He stated that a friend of ours was two blocks from the restaurant on 23rd Street. She was lying on the sidewalk, having a seizure, and asked whether we could come.

As we approached 8th Avenue, we saw the theater. There was an ambulance in front of it, but no Judy. I ran to the ambulance, and there she was, talking to the paramedics. From my understanding, her blood sugar levels had started to fall, and she fell in front of the theater. Some of the onlookers asked what they could do, and one of them went into the theater and got her a soda. The other spectator came and found us. All the paramedics could do was monitor her blood sugar and then let her go. We lost our reservations and had to eat at a dinner near the theater. I kept it to myself, but I was mad. It wasn't that she had a bad reaction that upset me; rather, it was the fact that she didn't take good care of herself in general. Even though we still made the show on time, her lack of self-care had still impacted us.

The next time I saw Judy have a diabetic seizure was when we were on a whitewater rafting trip to Pennsylvania. Judy's family had a house in the Pocono Mountains, which was located about thirty minutes from any hospital. On day 2, we were going to go paintballing. I woke up and started waking up the other people on the trip. I asked where Judy was. We eventually found her under some blankets in the living room. I shouted her name three times. She mumbled but was nonresponsive, but there was still hope. I took my blood testing kit out and tested her blood level. Her blood sugar was extremely low. Judy was about to go into a diabetic coma. We had no glucagon kit, and the nearest hospital was at least thirty minutes away.

I asked someone to find some honey. When they brought it to me, I stuck my finger in it and rubbed some on her lips. She started to lick her lips, so I continued to feed her. I once again called her name, and she responded but still mumbled. While continuing the process of putting honey on her lips, I went on talking to her. When she was responsive to her name and said, "What?" I asked her to sit up, and she did. I asked her to drink some orange juice and held the glass for her while she slowly started to drink it. Once she finished the orange juice, we needed to wait. I asked the others on the trip to leave her alone for a few minutes, and I left her to get some more orange juice.

When I got back to the living room, several people were moving her to the couch and she started throwing punches into the air. As I approached her to push the people away, I got hit in the process. At that point, she was on the couch, and I continued to talk her through it. I told her that everything would be all right, that she was in a safe place, and other things to calm her down. About ten minutes later, she said that she was sorry that she hit me. I told her not to worry about it and that I understood. I gave her the new glass of orange juice. She was now able to drink it on her own and was past the danger point. We then went paintballing. Judy came with us but took it easy by not participating in the paintball activities.

[We didn't call 911 first, but we should have, regardless of the time it would have taken for them to get there. They would have had a glucagon kit in the ambulance when they arrived. If I had been wrong, I would have wasted valuable time trying to revive my friend. If possible, using the glucagon kit with its premeasured dosage is the best solution for such a situation. If the individual with diabetes is responsive and can drink orange juice, let them drink some and have them test their blood again fifteen minutes later.

If the person with diabetes is not able to respond, use a glucagon kit (if you have one), and then call 911. That is the best and safest solution. If you don't have glucagon handy, it is always good to call 911 first if the person is nonresponsive so they are on the way before trying honey and so you don't waste time. If others are there to help you, get them to call while you start the process of testing the blood sugar level with a glucose meter.]

CHILD'S PERSPECTIVE

During these extreme low blood sugar events, I was consumed with extreme fright, along with lots of sadness and anger. The first one was still very scary, despite the kindness and comfort of my mom's friend

Tom. I didn't know what was going on as I was going in and out of consciousness. You think you are going to die and feel very ill. Your mind starts racing. Thoughts start to disappear the longer it goes on until you black out. I did feel comforted when Tom was carrying me. That helped to ease my fears.

The second low blood sugar episode was scary because I was more aware that the reaction was happening. I felt woozy, my legs felt like Jell-O, and my head was spinning. I was afraid to tell my mother because I didn't want her to get angry. The feelings came on about five minutes before it was time to leave for Disney World. I felt disoriented and confused, hoping it would just go away so the trip wouldn't get ruined. It didn't go away! As I lay down on the hotel bed, my mother asked whether I was feeling all right. I grudgingly gave in and told her that I didn't feel well and that my blood sugar might be low. My mother picked up the phone and called 911.

The next thing I remember is waking up in the hospital, scared and angry at the world and myself. I was embarrassed, but I was more scared that my mom would be angry with me and that I would be yelled at for ruining the trip. Even if she hadn't said it, I felt I had ruined everything, and I was even more furious that my diabetes was to blame. I felt that diabetes had ruined not only my life but also what could have been the best trip ever. I felt helpless and sad because I had less control over my life than when I was five years old, prior to getting this horrible disorder. The thought that everyone else that day just got up and went to the park spun in my head. I couldn't stop thinking about it while they rode all the rides that I had wanted to but couldn't because of this awful illness.

If I had told my mother about the low blood sugar sooner, I could have avoided the hospital altogether, but the frustration in my mother's body language and her tone of voice scared me more than the repercussions. It's hard to remember, but I may have allowed it to happen because of the sympathy I got after the first experience.

In the adult world, I kept seeing my mother's frustration and guilt around my disorder. It's very frustrating to have to stop all the time for blood tests, urine tests, reactions, and forgetting to take the kit with the insulin in it to the restaurant and having to go back to retrieve it. I was also burned out and tired at that point in my life from having to stop all the time to take care of this horrible illness. It was my denial that landed me in the hospital, as I couldn't see the consequences of my actions. Or I was just too young to understand the consequences of my actions. My age was part of the problem.

Not having my insulin wouldn't stop me from eating if I was at school or on my own. I would just eat and face the consequences later. That seemed like a better option than pissing Mom and Dad off. Sometimes when I went to McDonald's with my dad, I would lie and pretend to give my shot by going to the bathroom.

The first two diabetic seizures were a piece of cake compared to the last one. I felt lost in my room. I was angry with myself that I couldn't study, and my thoughts were becoming self-defeating: "I am so stupid and useless." I got angry at the book and threw it on the bed. I felt a rage come over me, and I didn't know what or where it came from. I got a grip on myself, went to the bed, picked up the book, and nearly fell over. After getting the book, I felt as if I were drunk and couldn't walk straight. My legs felt heavy. I managed to get the book onto my desk. Then I became very sleepy and said that I must be tired, so I went back over to the bed and lay down and fell asleep. I awoke and looked at the clock and thought it was 10:00 p.m. instead of 4:00 p.m. My mind and vision were blurry. I didn't think anything was wrong, but if it was 10:00 p.m., I needed to get ready for bed.

I stared at Larry and his girlfriend. I saw empty plates, and I was angry that they had eaten without me. My emotions were everywhere. I was having hallucinations and delusional thoughts. I felt paranoid and just wanted to hide. As I got upstairs, I felt great relief. The room appeared dark. The light wouldn't turn on, and I fell into bed. I felt great fear as I awoke to see two police officers trying to get me. I was scared and thought they were demons. I thought I was going to die.

In the hospital, I felt as if the devil had ripped my soul right out of me. I was drained, scared, and wouldn't let anyone touch me. For me, it was easier to accept the mental shift during a diabetic seizure as a child than as an adult.

PARENTAL ADVICE

This section refers to preventing diabetic seizure/coma.

Refer to table 3.1 in the "Clinical Advice" section of chapter 3 to identify what age is appropriate for self-monitoring. If your child is not old enough to be monitoring their own blood sugars, make sure you test their sugars first thing in the morning, before each shot/bolus, before eating, before meals, and before going to bed. In addition, have your child wear a CGM (continuous glucose monitor). It will reduce the chances of a seizure.

Be aware of how you emotionally react to your child when he/she forget to bring the insulin, blood testing kits, and other needed apparatus for managing diabetes. There is a saying that my mother would use a lot that is useful to remember: "Man plans, and God laughs." Plans need to be flexible, and your child's health is more important than arriving on time.

Living with diabetes is about living with unpredictability. If plans are not flexible, then frustration will follow. Continued frustration can cause your child to stop telling you when their blood sugar is low or high or when they eat without giving insulin. Parents need to understand that children learn through observation. If your children see you get upset after they have told you that they have forgotten to give their insulin, it may reduce the chances that they will tell you when it happens again. Getting emotional help for your child and yourself can open communication and reduce the emotional impact of living with such a difficult illness. Getting angry doesn't help. I know you are scared, but remember, so is your child. Avoid worrying about what will happen and address each incident in a calm and relaxed manner when things happen in the moment.

It is important to have you and your child attend counseling/psy-chotherapy sessions to manage the emotional issues that come with diabetes, including loss of freedom, isolation, guilt, sadness, frustration, anger, and other feelings that revolve around your child's diabetes or your own feelings of helplessness, guilt, anger, loss, and others. This will help you clear your head so signs of out-of-control blood sugars won't get overlooked. Psychotherapy for children and adults with diabetes is more than treating a psychiatric condition; it is for coping with your health condition. Having a release valve where you can express your feelings about an illness that comes with many harmful, self-abusive feelings is extremely valuable and can make a real difference in your child's management as well as his/her emotional well-being. Reducing your frustration and having someone to talk to about the daily trials and tribulations can improve your life as a parent too.

It is important to encourage your child to stop to check blood sugars. When a reaction comes, it is good to let your child know directly and indirectly that it is not only acceptable to stop and take care of their diabetes-related issues but also encouraged. You could say things such as "It's a nice place to stop for a break during a trip" and then have them check their blood sugar level, or after they say they need to check it or rest, you can say, "That's great because I needed to go to the bathroom anyway." Treat it as a rest break for the family and make the best of it. If you respond with comments of resistance like "Hurry up! We don't have time for this," or "We will be late!" then your child is less likely to let you know when a problem is happening. Keep in mind that if you are walking long distances, a snack will need to be given. This includes walking around the mall, shopping, going up and down aisles in the grocery store, and so on.

If your child is having a low blood sugar reaction, don't deviate from the fifteen-grams/fifteen-minutes rule (if after fifteen minutes the blood sugar level is still low, give another fifteen carbs). Glucose gel, tablets, or powder, as well as hard candy or another simple carbohydrate, is appropriate to give for a reaction. Do not use chocolate or any other complex carbohydrate to treat a low blood sugar reaction, as complex carbohydrates like cake work too slowly. It can mean the difference between getting back to normal and feeling better in fifteen minutes and struggling to get the blood sugar back in to a healthy range. When using low blood sugar as an excuse to eat sweets, people tend to give more carbs and continue to give even more carbs after fifteen minutes when the blood sugar hasn't changed. The original treat (carbs) could take up to sixty minutes to work. If you eat more while you are waiting for it to work, by the time you are back to feeling better, you may have already given too much and will spend the next four to six hours dealing with high blood sugars. It will feel like a yo-yo effect, going from low to high blood sugars and having to deal with each of them one after the other.

Once your child's blood sugar has stabilized, you may occasionally reward your child with a special treat. Let them know it is important that they don't use other sweets to handle a low blood sugar reaction. Depending on your wishes and the given situation, tell them that it is okay to have a treat from time to time as long as insulin is given for it. You could also reward them for catching the reaction before it got too bad with a treat once in a while. Give them plenty of positive feedback, and show them that it is okay to take care of themselves and their diabetes. Be flexible with keeping schedules and reinforce that it is okay to be late somewhere in order to take care of their needs.

Avoid frustration when your child has to use the restroom every hour on a road trip, and don't yell at them for something diabetes-related like high blood sugar, as even adults struggle to get management right. Instead, remember that high blood sugar may be causing frequent urinations. Ask them to check their blood sugar in a calm and comforting voice. When traveling, keep in mind that extra insulin will be needed if your child is going to be confined to sitting for hours on end. During my childhood, I spent many trips holding my bladder to the point of pain before asking my dad to pull over. The more frustrated you are with the daily challenges of having diabetes, the more your kid is going to see taking care of themselves, like speaking up or testing blood sugars, as negative.

As a child, I saw speaking up as negative. Many times, I said nothing and lived with blood sugars that had to be in the 300s. On the trip with my mom, I was afraid to tell her that there was a problem. I recall taking a test and seeing that my blood sugar was a little low a half hour before my seizure in Florida. I didn't tell her because I didn't want to upset her. This decision led to not telling her sooner that I was feeling bad and that my blood sugar was low, which created the consequence of going to the hospital.

Contact a therapist who specializes in diabetes or chronic illness. They will help you and your family with the emotional impact of diabetes. The more flexible and understanding you are around change and the more you focus on the positive things your child is doing, such as good grades in school, making the baseball team, and taking care of their diabetes, the more they will come to you for help when they need it. Understand that it is normal for blood sugars to fluctuate. Blood sugars are not good or bad; they are just information that gives us clues about what to do next. Sometimes it is high (wait until insulin on board is done or give insulin as needed) and sometimes it is low (fifteen-carb snack if no insulin is on board and it is above 60 mg/dL, or fifteen carbs of glucose if below 60mg/dL), but no matter what it is, remember to be accepting of it and encourage better management instead of reprimanding your child for being human.

CLINICAL ADVICE

The following factors can lead to a diabetic seizure/coma.

Hypoglycemia: Your brain needs glucose to function. In severe cases, low blood sugar may cause you to pass out. Hypoglycemia is most common in people who take too much insulin or skip meals or snacks. Exercising too vigorously or drinking too much alcohol can have the same effect. How quickly your blood sugar drops influences the symptoms of hypoglycemia. For example, if it takes a few hours for your blood sugar to drop 50 mg/dL (3 mmol/L), the symptoms may be minimal. If your blood sugar drops the same amount in a few minutes, the symptoms will be more pronounced (source: Mayo Clinic under health/diabetic/coma).

What is a *hypoglycemic diabetic seizure*? It starts with a hypoglycemic episode including weak, shaky muscles similar to alcohol withdrawal for an alcoholic. If it goes untreated, your muscles will start to tremor. Eventually it becomes uncontrollable, and it will be difficult, even next to impossible, to treat the low blood sugar reaction yourself. If you don't get outside help from your family, friends, or medical professionals and they don't render assistance, what started as being a little shaky will turn into a diabetic seizure. Prior to the seizure, there are signs and symptoms to prevent it. Since it progresses slowly most of the time, there is usually plenty of opportunity to stop the seizure. When it is left untreated, glucose levels in the brain continue to reduce and the brain's ability to function properly decreases. Since the brain's main food is glucose, when it is taken away, the brain starts to shut down and the seizure starts to happen, leading to unconsciousness.

This unconsciousness is a *diabetic coma*. It is a state of unconsciousness similar to a coma one might get from a concussion. While in this state, you can't be awakened or respond consciously to visual stimuli. There is minimal (if any) reaction to sounds or other types of stimulation.

Prolonged hypoglycemia-induced comas can lead to brain damage. Multiple, extended periods of time in an extreme hypoglycemia state (several hours untreated) can cause memory loss and other cognitive issues. I have seen this problem when working with clients who have had multiple comas a month for several years. If glucagon is administered quickly, it is unlikely that any noticeable damage will occur. This is why it is important to check blood sugars often. It is also helpful to set your glucose level goal a little higher during the night, while you sleep—about 10–20 mg/dL higher. Please consult with your endocrinologist or CDE (certified diabetes educator) for guidance around setting nighttime basal rates and before making any changes to your diabetes management.

A hypoglycemic diabetic coma is avoidable through managing your diabetes by using a continuous glucose monitor and paying attention to low blood sugar symptoms, including:

- Feeling weak
- Tiredness
- Increased sweating
- Moderate to extreme levels of hunger
- Irritability
- Unstable emotions
- Confusion

The causes of *hyperglycemic diabetic comas* are prolonged blood sugar extremes, which cause various conditions.

Ketoacidosis: If your muscle cells become starved for energy, your body may respond by breaking down fat stores. This process forms toxic acids known as ketones. Left untreated, ketoacidosis can lead to a diabetic coma. Ketoacidosis is most common in people who have type 1 diabetes, but it can also affect people who have type 2 diabetes or gestational diabetes (source: Mayo Clinic under health/diabetic/coma).

Hyperosmolar syndrome: If your blood sugar level tops 600 milligrams per deciliter (mg/dL), or 33 millimoles per liter (mmol/L), this condition is known as hyperosmolar syndrome. When your blood sugar gets this high, your blood becomes thick and syrupy. The excess sugar passes from your blood into your urine, which triggers a filtering process that draws tremendous amounts of fluid from your body. Left untreated, hyperosmolar syndrome can cause life-threatening dehydration and loss of consciousness. Hyperosmolar syndrome is most common in older adults who have type 2 diabetes (source: Mayo Clinic under health/diabetic/coma).

A hyperglycemic coma is avoidable through managing your diabetes, using a continuous glucose monitor, and paying attention to high blood sugar symptoms, including:

- Increased thirst
- Frequent urination
- Cotton mouth
- Dry skin
- Dry and irritated eyes
- Nausea
- Vomiting
- Shortness of breath
- Feeling lethargic
- Poor memory
- Feeling depressed
- Overemotionality

The resulting diabetic coma from any of the above causes requires medical help and is serious enough to call 911. Left untreated for extended periods of time, it can lead to death or brain damage.

If you can't wake up the person living with diabetes, don't hesitate to call 911. Test blood sugars second. If low, try honey. What I did by not calling 911 reflected inexperience. In the future, if I am in that type of situation again, I won't hesitate to call 911 first with my friend's or child's life on the line. The honey and juice are to prevent coma. In situations when it doesn't work, you haven't wasted time, because you already called 911.

8

Navigating High Blood Sugar Hell!

THURSDAY, JULY 16, 1987

Terry was diagnosed during the summer before entering third grade and became depressed shortly after. Despite the doctor's warnings that high blood sugars can lead to neuropathy and other issues later in life, he still cheated. He could have gone into diabetes ketoacidosis or worse multiple times throughout childhood. As a result of having to manage a difficult disorder and blood-sugar-related depression, he became chronically depressed. At twelve years old, Terry was suicidal. Sorry, I am getting ahead of myself once again.

Terry was having trouble reading and writing as he entered third grade. After taking some tests, the school decided to put him into "Mr. Kotter's" classroom (the name is from a class of low achievers from a television sitcom that ran from 1975 to 1979). Terry was no Arnold Horshack (a character from the show) or any of the other Sweathogs, but he felt like it and isolated himself from the other kids.

A few weeks after the start of the third grade, they called his mother and told her to come into school. While sitting in the principal's office, in a seat Terry would get very used to over those few years, the principal explained that there was a problem with his reading and writing, and they (the principal, the vice principal, and the school counselor) recommended a place to get tested.

As Terry walked out of that meeting, it looked as if his daydreaming was coming to an end. He looked at his mother, and she was mad. Terry can still remember the look on her face as the principal told her of their concerns. He was scared because he felt that it was his fault. On the drive back from school, there was silence in the car for most of the ride home. Once they got home, his mom called his father at work. As Terry recalled, he agreed with the school's recommendation, and a week later his mom and dad took off from work and drove him to get tested at the Kingsbury Center for learning disabilities in Washington, D.C.

They got there around 10:00 a.m. and waited in the lobby to be seen as his father filled out the paperwork. On arrival, Terry asked where the bathroom was. He went right to it and took what seemed like the longest pee yet. Like most long trips, he had held it in for most of the journey. It was a game for him to see how long he could go without using the bathroom and how long he would piss. The longer the peeing, the prouder of his stamina he became. After taking a very satisfying pee, Terry went to sit in the waiting room with his mother. The social worker introduced herself as the counselor who would be spending time with him while he took a few tests. She was very nice. Terry remembered liking her.

Terry remembered the layout as it centered on the bathroom. He had a visual memory of the bathroom but little of the rest of the building. Terry could not tell you how to get there or which office belonged to his counselor, whom he saw multiple times, but he could tell you where the bathroom was and describe it in excruciating detail. The same went for every location Terry was at for any length of time. Going to the bathroom a lot is a sure sign of high blood sugar.

Terry spent what felt like forever there, taking the many tests. These tests included WISC-R, Bender-Gestalt, the Slingerland Screening Test for identifying children with specific language disabilities, the Gray Oral Reading Test, Wepman's™ Auditory Discrimination Test, Wide Range Achievement Test, the Temple University Informal Reading Inventory, and other informal observation tests. After a long day of testing, he was diagnosed with a learning disorder and having the symptoms that could be related to dyslexia. Terry had problems in sound blending, oral reading, some perceptual tasks, spelling, and the mechanics of writing. The implied diagnosis given on January 28, 1991, was a reading comprehension disorder and that he had phonological processing problems common in dyslexia. Terry didn't understand what this meant as a child, but he knew one thing for sure: the gap between him and the other kids was larger than ever before.

"What were my blood sugars that day?" Terry asks himself that a lot when he thinks about that day. He remembers many days sitting in class and going to the bathroom over and over again. Terry couldn't focus on school work and spent the time daydreaming that he was James Bond. No one made the connection. Many bathroom visits during a period of school meant that he had high blood sugar, which he eventually figured out, though it didn't stop his cheating.

During the testing, Terry remembers having trouble concentrating while he was fixated on his need to go to the bathroom, instead of on the test. He remembers thinking how his bladder hurt and wondering when he would get a break to relieve himself. He waited more than a half hour before asking whether he could use the restroom. Having to pee a lot was common for Terry, and during that half hour he didn't recall anything except having to urinate. Terry went to the bathroom at every break. He was always smart and creative, but he just didn't get grammar or phonics. So how did Terry get to this point?

Terry had high blood sugars during the day, but when he went home, he would correct his sugars by giving himself a shot. Terry always checked his sugar levels when he got home, and they were almost always high. Terry didn't want his mom to find out, so he gave a shot, and after an hour or two, his blood sugars would be in range. Every now and then, his mom would get home and ask him to test. He would always have normal blood sugars by then.

Blood sugar plays a role in all areas of focus and concentration. High or low blood sugar can cause test results to be of one's physical state instead of one's knowledge of the material. Maybe Terry could read fine when he was being evaluated, but at the time they tested him, his blood sugar was very high, so this hurt his ability to read. He recalls not feeling well most of his childhood. Terry was unusually tired, had nausea, and went to the bathroom one to two times an hour. When his blood sugar wasn't high, Terry would go only one or two times a day.

Terry's blood sugar could have been tested three times a day and adjusted with insulin during his school day, but it wasn't. No one had thought about it back then. The better control a child has over his diabetes, the higher the chance that he will have a better prognosis and minimize the impact on his developing brain.

So no one caught it, and Terry didn't blame anyone, except maybe himself at times. He knew enough to recognize the negative impacts of out-of-control blood sugars. Who would know to test one's blood sugar level before a test or class in the 1990s or even now, unless a parent knows and points it out to the school? Before Terry left the specialist's office, he was told that he would have to study harder as well as be tutored in spelling and reading three times a week. They told his parents that tutoring would give him the necessary tools to process information and understand various aspects of reading and writing so he could follow along in class. So for the next three to four years, Terry was tutored in English.

Terry didn't have control of his blood sugars until high school, and by then he had multiple cognitive issues. He was put in special education from third to ninth grade with a diagnosis of dyslexia and a reading disorder. Having erratic blood sugar levels throughout early childhood caused his brain to develop with an imbalance. Terry had learned to live with it. Being overly prepared for class helped his preparation for life itself. He worked harder in the moment, so if his blood sugars were high, he had time to wait for blood sugars to return to normal before studying. By doing that, he reduced the struggle of learning, but during class he still had problems.

DEPRESSION

Depression sets in early in life for many children with diabetes due to many factors, and it did for Terry. Looking back now, Terry knows when it started. It started with anger shortly after being told he wasn't allowed to have cake for his ninth birthday. Other factors contributed to his depression. This included the isolation of living with diabetes and poor blood sugar control, which was mostly high. Terry doesn't recall much happiness from ages eight to sixteen years old. Depression played a big part in his poor memory and lack of happiness, but it was the high blood sugars that contributed to his increasing levels of depression during that period.

SIXTEEN TO SEVENTY AND PICKING UP SPEED

Terry was sixteen years old at the time, and he was in his car driving. He was heading away from his home as he made a left turn onto a very winding road. Without thinking, he hit the gas hard and was up to 70 miles per hour by the time he came to the wheat (weed) field where he had planned to end his life. Terry turned the wheel hard right and headed toward a tree. The car bounced all over the place. He missed the tree by inches and came to a halt. Terry got out of the car and lay in the field, watching the puffy clouds go by. He thought how funny it was and laughed to himself. The universe wouldn't let him kill himself—go figure. "Luck favored the foolish," he said.

Terry lay there laughing to himself for an hour or so; then he got up and drove back home. He was happy, and he thought it was the first happiness he had ever felt. The funny thing was, as he looked back on all those years leading up to this event, Terry couldn't remember being happy. With poor blood sugar management came poor memory, diminished ability to learn, and depression. Life was just a fog for Terry.

The more he talked about this situation in session, he started to see some brief glimpses of happiness from that period of his life.

At some point during his late twenties, Terry viewed an old 8 mm film his father had taken prior to his diabetes diagnosis, from birth until he was about six years old. He was so excited that there was actual proof of happiness in his life! Terry watched himself playing with his father, enjoying several of his birthday parties (with sugar-filled cakes and clowns), swimming at the beach, and bowling.

After laughing to himself on the day of his suicide attempt, most of the rest of that afternoon was a blur. He just remembers the drive home and being thankful that no one saw him or knew he had tried. Terry was so embarrassed. He went to bed as normal that day and had a dream that was so real he was compelled to tell about it. In session, and with crystal clear detail, he shared that dream as if he had just awakened.

In the dream, Terry was twelve again, trying to kill himself. Terry was on the balcony of the apartment he used to live in. He was talking to a mirror image of himself. "We were on the balcony of my old apartment. I grabbed the other me, this clone, and we started to struggle. It seemed like we struggled for hours. Eventually, I threw the clone off the balcony and watched as the clone fell to his death." Terry felt lucky it wasn't him. He said he no longer wanted to die and would fight to stay alive. He killed his clone (the depression) that night.

THE NURSE MESSES UP

The day after his suicide attempt, Terry got ready for school and took the bus. He felt happy and wanted to tell someone. Terry was having a low blood sugar reaction and went to the school nurse to get juice he kept in her refrigerator. He started to tell her his dream as she went to get his juice. He told her that he didn't want to kill himself anymore because of his dream.

Later that day, Terry was called to the counselor's office. He met with her, and she told him that everyone was worried. She informed him that the principal and vice principal were in a meeting with his teachers to figure out what to do. Terry started laughing so hard that his ribs hurt. He laughed for what seemed like an hour, but in reality it was only ten minutes.

After his outburst, Terry told the social worker that the nurse had messed up. He said, "I wasn't going to kill myself. I was talking about a dream." He described the dream and told her that he finally felt good after all these years. She wondered why he was laughing at such a serious time while everyone was worried about him. Terry explained how ridiculous it was that all the times he thought of killing himself (and even tried), no one at school had noticed. Now that he was free of that burden, every member of the school staff was meeting to make sure he was safe. Terry laughed all the way back to art class.

SUICIDE OR COMFORT!

What Terry was going through is common for children with diabetes who don't have proper supports in place. Not understanding what was happening to him brought Terry to the brink of insanity, and thoughts of suicide brought him comfort. His first suicidal thoughts were at twelve years old. Terry said it was scary but comforting at the same time. On his first attempt, he struggled to kill himself. He stayed awake for twenty-four hours. Terry lay on his bed with a hunting knife held to his wrist, which he had bought in an army surplus store two years earlier at ten years old. Terry was rubbing the knife up and down his wrist. Redness started to appear.

Terry's mind was spinning with several thoughts: "When is Mom going to look to see if I am okay? Is she going to even look? Not that she cares about me! She never did." Terry's mind continued: "No one cares!" and "I will show her!" One thought prevented him from changing the direction of the knife and slicing his wrists open: "You can't do this to your father." It was followed by "You're all alone and no one cares; your mother didn't even come to see where you were!" These two thoughts played over and over again in his head. Like a roulette wheel that eventually landed on the winning number, he chose his father. He got up crying, knife in hand, and asked his mother, "Why didn't you come and see if I was okay?" followed by "You don't care! I could have killed myself and you wouldn't care!" After this attempt to kill himself, his mother found him a child psychologist, whom he saw for a year or two.

DYING INSIDE AND OUT

Terry focused on every negative thing in his life. Before the first suicide attempt when he was twelve years old, he had thought of several ways he could kill himself. Terry loved looking over the balcony, the same balcony that was in his dream. While he was living at that apartment, he would often go out onto the balcony. Terry only went out on the balcony to imagine how he was going to kill himself. He would watch the stuck-up women walking their dogs in the garden below. He would say, "I hate them, walking their dogs in their perfect lives" and "I will show them." As Terry.watched them, his imagination would take over and he visualized getting up on the railing, jumping off, and then silently falling until he hit bottom.

Sometimes he imagined that one of the dog walkers would look up and scream as Terry fell. In his mind, a smile always came to his face just before he hit the pavement. Other times, Terry would be falling and he would wake out of his fantasy. During this time in his life, Terry liked thinking this way. This fantasy was the only thing that made him happy, as he was comforted by the knowledge that he could escape his diabetes once and for all.

One time he even sat on the rail of the balcony and thought of pushing off, doing a back flip to his death to end the pain. There were many dark times during the eight years of his depression. Terry thought suicide was an answer to his pain.

As Terry got older, he had several thoughts around death and started collecting knives. He even bought a 22 mm handgun through mail order. Terry liked having these things around to ease his pain. He was never a cutter, but he liked the comfort of knowing he could protect himself from even more pain than he already had.

TERRY FINALLY GOT IT!
After his last suicide attempt at sixteen years old, he started taking care of himself. For the first time, he made real attempts to manage his diabetes. Terry went back to therapy for two years, and everything got progressively better. The more he managed his blood sugars, the better he felt; the better he felt, the easier it became to manage diabetes, and so on. Over time, the cloud lifted while clarity and control took over.

Before going off to college, Terry had started to take his diabetes seriously. He was monitoring his blood sugars and tested more often. During college, Terry knew he could ask for reasonable accommodations, but did he want them? No, he didn't. He didn't want to be singled out. Extra time would have helped in college, but it was going to be a new life for him. After college, he managed to get himself to New York City to follow his dream of becoming a famous artist. His passion for the arts took him around the world. At one point, he even learned to speak Japanese for his show in Japan. Terry had to take several classes over, but he learned enough to communicate at the art exhibition, which gave him the confidence to go back to school.

Terry was in the process of looking at schools and studying for his GRE when his best friend at the time had introduced him to his future wife, Maya. They went out to an Korean restaurant for dinner. As they said goodbye that evening, he grabbed her passionately and they had the most romantic kiss ever. The rest was history. His self-esteem was low when he met her, but she seemed to complete him.

Maya recognized that Terry had ADD and informed him that he could get reasonable accommodations on the GRE if he got tested. He later learned you could also get it for diabetes. Upon the recommendation of his wife, he was retested so he could get special accommodations for his learning disabilities. Terry asked his general practitioner whether she knew of any good neuropsychologists, and she referred him to

Dr. Thomas in Manhattan. Terry scheduled an appointment with Dr. Thomas, who rediagnosed him. As an adult, he was now stuck with a diagnosis of depression NOS/dysthyma (a low-level depression) and attention deficit disorder. He went several times and took many psychological tests. Terry made sure that every time he went in for testing, his blood sugar was normal.

Dr. Thomas referred him to a psychiatrist who put him on a stimulant to help his focus. His childhood memories came back, some good and some bad, but he was glad to have them. It wasn't perfect, but after a year of trial and error, he is now on a combination of medication that works best for him. Thanks to the new medications, Terry's life began to change for the better and his diabetes management improved tenfold.

CHILD'S PERSPECTIVE
The following section is on ADD, learning disorders, and depression.

Terry was not really sure how he felt about the learning disorders due to the depression. After some reflection, there were some things he related to the learning issues, as not all issues come from diabetes. Terry saw the learning disorders as another flaw, difference, and an abnormal part of him that once again isolated him from the other children. He was angry with his parents and himself for not protecting him from this. Terry was uninformed about why he had the disabilities and what was going to happen with him. This caused him to feel lost and alone.

Depression caused many problems in his life. Like many children, Terry felt alone with his diabetes and scared. He felt like a loser and stupid that he couldn't accomplish and remember what other kids could easily do. He blamed himself for his problems with phonics, sugar levels, and just about any other problem that came along. Terry would say to himself, "You're a loser," all the time. He blamed himself for the cheating that caused the high blood sugars. Terry would feel bad and depressed about eating a bag of candy, which caused him to have problems living up to his responsibilities. Terry didn't realize that he was still a child and that it was okay to not be perfect.

Terry took on adult responsibilities but lacked the coping skills needed to address and deal with the adult responsibility. He would be very hard on himself and felt he was a disappointment to his parents, which is common among all kids when their parents expect something of them and they aren't able to do it.

Terry felt caught between being a child and being an adult. He wanted to be like other kids, but the reality is that Terry couldn't be like them, as he was supposed to say no to sweets when offered. In his attempts to fit in, he said yes, disregarding his diabetes and health. How he went about fitting in was making his life worse. Terry even knew at one point what the high blood sugars were doing, but he didn't care. In children (and adults) with diabetes, high blood sugars make the world around them distorted and out of focus. But despite that, in an effort to fit in, Terry would eat fast food or cake at a birthday party even if he didn't have insulin to take. Terry felt he had to always be normal. He would not say, "I can't eat now because I forgot my shot," or "We have to go back to get it," because he would stand out like a sore thumb.

Most kids will do anything to fit in, and Terry was no different. Whether he forgot his shot or not, if his parents asked whether he had taken his shot, the answer was always yes.

Since Terry felt having diabetes was his fault, he wouldn't tell his parents if he forgot to bring his shot when they went out for dinner. He didn't want to burden them any more than he already had while being blamed and yelled at. Terry was sad a lot during the depression and disconnected from the world. He saw people around him, but they were not part of his world. Terry felt they couldn't understand what it was like for him as an outcast from his peers to be different. The weight of the world is very difficult for adults to carry alone, but for young children with diabetes, it is unbearable. The emotional isolation from other children when standing in the cafeteria filled with other children eating whatever they want becomes overwhelming.

PARENTAL ADVICE

My best advice is to work as a team with your child and other family members to reduce your child's heavy feeling around living with diabetes. Brainstorm with your child to find solutions that work for you both and that help them take care of their diabetes and other physical and mental issues:

1. Carry an extra blood testing kit with a shot and insulin with you in case your child or teenager forgets. That way, when your child forgets to bring their kit, you don't have to return home to fix the problem.
2. Teach your child age-appropriate tasks of diabetes management (see the "Clinical Advice" section of chapter 3).
3. Help your child with the process of managing their diabetes.
4. Have your children test blood sugar levels several times during school.
5. Remain in touch with the school teachers and administration (see the "Parental Advice" section of chapter 9), and instruct them on how you want them to help your child. Make sure that your child takes part in creating the school plan and agrees with it.
6. Let your child know it is okay to reach out to you, regardless of the issue. Tell them you won't get mad. Then follow through if they come to you, discuss the problem with them, remain calm, be the adult, and be understanding.
7. Discuss the cause of the problem and discuss how to solve it as a team.
8. Teach your child that it is important to love himself or herself, regardless of other people's opinions.
9. Talk to your child regularly about their feelings.
10. Listen to your child and adjust to his or her needs, but continue to maintain the existing healthy boundaries (rules) that exist for their safety.

11. Spend time doing fun things (your children like to do) with them weekly (i.e., play video games with them, go camping, fishing, etc.).

12. Don't forget to have fun. Life can be full of fun and games as well as responsibility.

13. Stay away from labeling your child as sick. Your children are capable of living a long and full, healthy life.

14. As parents, you need to reach out for help. If you don't take care of you first, how can you be there for your children?

15. It is not your fault or your children's fault. It just is.

16. Get second opinions.

17. Advocate for your children, and teach your children to advocate for themselves.

18. Create balance between taking care of your children and letting them take care of themselves.

19. Asking "How was your day?" when your child gets home from school does not leave room for elaboration and health discussions. Instead, try "What did you do at school today?" as it leaves plenty of room for discussions to occur naturally. Stay away from questions where the answer is good/bad, yes/no, and other questions that only have one-word answers.

20. Try starting your questions with "What?" Have a discussion about what happened by asking:
    A. What did you do in or during . . . ?
    B. Who (followed by "What" or "Why" statement) did you eat lunch with?
       a. What did you talk about?
       b. Why did you eat lunch with John? I thought you didn't like him.
    C. How (followed by "What" or "Why" statement) did you feel today?
       a. What made you feel that way?
       b. Why did you feel that way?

21. Let your child know it is okay to feel their feelings (i.e., sad, angry, depressed, etc.). If they do, your child could talk to you or other

supportive members of the family about why they are feeling that way. (A lot of the time, even if you do everything right, your child still may not want to talk. A good therapist can help with that.)

22. To help with everything above:
    A. Individual therapy for both you and your children that includes family sessions (preferably one familiar with diabetes or chronic illness)
    B. Certified diabetes educators
    C. Family therapy
    D. Diabetes clinics like the Friedman Diabetes Institute in New York City
    E. Diabetes organizations like Juvenile Diabetes Foundation
    F. Your child's endocrinologist
    G. Parenting groups

CLINICAL ADVICE

This section is on factors that impact the brain's development that may cause psychiatric issues and takes a look at long-term consequences of poorly managed blood sugar levels.

There are several factors that play a role in your child's mental health. Emotional energy transmissions, chemical adaptation, and age of onset are factors that put your child at risk for future complications. The last and most important factor (because it can be managed) is diabetes management, which impacts the development of the brain and other long-term consequences. Most of these factors can be resolved to give your child the best shot at a long and healthy life.

Emotions

To gain a full understanding of the causes of psychiatric issues, we need to look at factors that impact the brain's development. Emotional energy transmissions and chemical adaptation are important in understanding how clinical depression and other psychiatric disabilities are formed in children. The last influence is the physical and chemical changes during the development of the brain.

What Are Emotional Energy Transmissions?

So imagine you are in a great mood, sitting on the couch and watching television, and you just made partner at the firm you work at. You are eagerly awaiting the return of your significant other to tell him the good news.

Your significant other bursts through the door angry, doesn't say a word, walks right by you, and heads into the kitchen. You feel tense, and the happiness dissipates as you feel a sense of dread. His intense emotions radiate from across the room, impacting your emotions. You wait anxiously for him to come out of the kitchen. The anxious feeling is so tense that you can't stand it, and now you are angry.

This happens because of emotional energy transmissions due to psychic energy, which is energy or emotional moods stored in the solar plexus that radiates out and gets transferred to those around them. Bioelectrography studies these electric emissions of living organisms. It focuses on measuring fields of physical, emotional, mental, and spiritual energy emanating to and from an individual as well as plants or inanimate objects.

Freud referred to the process of releasing instinctual energy as catharsis (meaning to purge or cleanse). It is the release of emotions and tensions. Therapy techniques like psychodrama and primal scream therapy have used cathartic experiences to help people heal in a controlled environment. In uncontrolled environments, this energy released as anger and other heavy emotions can impact those around them, even if the people are not interacting with the individual who is angry or even know them (i.e., a stranger on the bus sitting next to you).

Chemical Adaptation

Emotional energy transmissions and the behavior of people within their environment will affect a child's development. Their brain chemistry will balance to match a child's environment due to the human body's unique ability to adapt for survival. Unfortunately, that same survival mode of the human body, the ability to adjust brain chemistry in order to adapt to one's environment, is one of the causes of chemical imbalances that lead to psychiatric disorders.

A child's first environment is a mother's womb, where nonpsychic emotional energy transmission happens between mother and child. During pregnancy, depression is not learned but felt by the baby through the mother. The baby feels what the mother feels. The baby adapts chemically and developmentally to living with the mother's emotions. If the mother is depressed throughout her pregnancy, the child will be more prone to depression than someone whose mother had healthy emotions during pregnancy.

The mind, emotion, and body connection are powerful factors on the development of a child. I am not saying that prenatal babies or even young children are clinically depressed—merely that all, including depressed or intense, emotions are transmitted and absorbed by the children in a family during the developmental stages of life.

Children who grow up in negative environments are more likely to develop depression or other psychiatric issues than children growing up in an emotionally balanced environment. If after the birth the mother is no longer depressed and the parents are emotionally stable, the brain chemistry will return to normal. The brain will repair itself, and the child will develop in a healthy fashion.

For children with diabetes, the consequences of a negative environment are highly problematic. For example, a child with a normal blood sugar level is in the room during a fight between you and your partner. The anger in the room causes a negative emotional state in your child, who wasn't originally upset to begin with. This causes your child's body to release cortisol (glucose) into the bloodstream. As the negative emotional state continues in your child and their environment, cortisol continues to be secreted by the adrenal glands to assist in managing stressful events. This hormone is believed to be related to clinical depression, but any negative emotional state may release it into the blood system, causing high blood sugar levels. Should your child encounter a negative environment, it is important to keep a close eye on their blood sugar levels.

Very few people account for this context in their management of blood glucose levels because it is a relatively unpredictable variable that impacts one's blood sugar levels negatively. The best you can do is be aware, and during stressful or depressed days, test more often. Pay attention to how negative environments impact your child's blood sugar levels. Understand that chronic depression is formed during the development period of the brain from conception to age eighteen years old. As a parent, you need to be aware of how unhealthy behavior and negative environments impact your children and their development.

Age of Onset

Age of onset's role in future problems means that the earlier one develops diabetes, the higher the risk for future psychiatric complications due primarily to physical and chemical adaptation as well as frontal lobe scarring caused by extreme high, low, and uncontrolled blood sugar levels. I feel it is important as a diabetes-focused psychotherapist to help all parents understand how and what causes emotional problems in their children in order to help with prevention.

Age of onset means the younger the child, the less ability a child has to take responsibility for maintaining proper blood sugar levels. The less developed a child is, the more pliable the brain. Therefore, any kind of trauma including ill health can lead to lasting behavioral and cognitive deficits later in life. So basically a four-year-old with a HbA1c of 9 will cause significantly more damage to the developing brain than a ten-year-old with the same A1c of 9.

So, how do high or low blood sugar levels impact the human brain?

High sugars: Well, imagine you are trying to make gravy and you use double the required flour that the recipe calls for. It becomes so thick that it no longer pours out of the gravy boat, so the gravy can't get to the mashed potatoes or the turkey. The more sugar you have in your bloodstream, the thicker it becomes, just like flour to gravy. It thickens, causing the heart to push harder to circulate the blood. The rate of blood flow slows down, getting less oxygen to your extremities and brain. This causes poor circulation, which can lead to nerve damage to various parts of the body including the neuron and chemical synapses in the thought-processing center of the human brain.

Chemical synapses are specialized junctions through which neurons signal to each other. They allow neurons to form circuits in the central nervous system. They are essential to the biological calculations that form perception and thought. They permit the nervous system to interact with and control other systems within the human body.

A neuron is an edgy cell in the nervous system, which processes and transmits data by electrochemical signaling. Neurons are necessary components of the brain that create conscious thought. They respond to stimulus, which then informs the central nervous system of the presence of the stimuli. After processing the data, the neuron sends a response to the other areas of the body.

When sugar levels are high, blood thickening occurs, which causes a reduction of oxygen in the brain. This lessens responses to stimuli, and in turn chemical synapses don't function properly, reducing the brain's ability to process information and making it harder to think and process data clearly. It impacts memory recall, attention, concentration, focus, and retention of external information, making learning difficult and in some cases impossible for the child or adult with diabetes. It hinders the growth of new cells in the brain and body. During high blood sugar levels, the body has a harder time fighting off infection by reducing the strength of the white blood cells to attack foreign antibodies in the bloodstream.

Low blood sugars: Low glucose causes your blood to thin. Your heart rate increases, and the level of oxygen in your blood also increases significantly, which impacts the brain. It hinders the ability to think at just about any level. During low blood sugar levels, the mind and body lose control. The lower the blood glucose, the less control a person has mentally, physically, and emotionally.

Imagine playing tennis, with the ball representing the neurotransmitter molecules that are supposed to pass through synapses to the receptor site for information to be processed. In tennis, the synapses are represented by the court, the receptor sites are targets on the opposite side of the court, and the tennis balls are the molecules filled with the information needed to pass data along to the targets on the other side of the net. With normal blood sugars, you are playing in perfect weather. The courts are dry, and you serve the ball (information molecules). It goes over the net onto the court (information passes through the synapses) and then hits the target (receptor that receives the information) you were aiming for.

Same scenario now, but low blood sugars place the court on top of an ice rink (solid ice, very slippery). Serve 1, you fall on the ice and the ball (information molecules) doesn't get over the net. Love serving 15. Serve 2, you slip as you are serving and you fault on the serve. Serve 3, you fault again and lose a point. Love serving 30. Serve 4, you don't fault, but the ball (information molecules) can't bounce right and misses the target (receptor that receives the information).

The wind has picked up. It's now snowing and your blood sugar is at 30 mg/dL. You can't even get the ball (information molecules) in the air to serve (to start their journey to the receptors). The information never reaches the synapses or the targets. *Long-term complications develop gradually over time. They may eventually become disabling or life-threatening.*

Blood vessel and heart disease: There is a dramatic increase for those living with diabetes of getting various cardiovascular issues, including heart attack, stroke, coronary artery disease, atherosclerosis (narrowing of the arteries), and high blood pressure. About 75 percent of individuals with diabetes (those without good blood glucose control) will die of heart or blood vessel issues, according to the American Heart Association.

Nerve damage: Rapidly changing and excess levels of sugar will injure capillaries, the tiny blood vessels that provide nourishment to nerve endings. The most common area of the body for this to occur is in the legs, causing tingling, numbness, burning, or pain that begins in the toes and fingers. Over several months, the nerve damage spreads upward. If left untreated, a person can lose feeling in the affected limbs over the next few years. Nerve damage in the digestive track will cause problems as well. Symptoms are one or a combination of vomiting, diarrhea, constipation, or nausea. For men and women, sexual arousal and feeling in pleasure areas of the body may decrease, including erectile dysfunction for men.

Kidney damage (nephropathy): Uncontrolled blood sugar levels can damage millions of tiny blood vessel clusters that filter waste from your blood. This damage may lead to kidney disease, requiring the person with diabetes to start dialysis, or they may need to receive a kidney transplant.

Eye damage: The blood vessels in the retina can be damaged, called diabetic retinopathy. If untreated, this condition will lead to blindness. There are higher risks for problems, such as glaucoma and cataracts.

Foot damage: Nerve damage to the feet and/or poor blood circulation increases the risk of foot complications. If left untreated, minor injuries such as cuts and blisters may become serious infections. This damage can require amputation of the toe, foot, or even leg.

Skin and mouth conditions: Poor management of your diabetes may leave you susceptible to skin issues such as bacterial and fungal infections. Poor management of diabetes and dental hygiene can lead to gum infections.

Osteoporosis: Poor management of your diabetes may cause low bone mineral density, increasing the risk of osteoporosis.

9

Addressing the Problems at School

WEDNESDAY, APRIL 17, 1991

What a great day! "It's going to be the best day ever!" Terry could just feel it. With spring in the air, it felt great on his walk to school. Seventh grade would be coming to an end soon, and he couldn't wait until summer time. So let me catch you up: During seventh grade, Terry got to spend a lot of time with the vice principal of his school, thanks to several kids who liked to pick on him in physical education class. Terry would say this had happened more than ten times so far that year. Needless to say, he got into a lot of fights, and, believe it or not, Terry would win the physical fight but lose because it always looked like he was the one who started the fight. Oh, well, he had made it through physical education class without fighting today. It was going to be a great day.

THIRD PERIOD

Now Terry was in one of his favorite classes: art class. It was someone's birthday today, and he brought cupcakes, compliments of his mother— Terry was sure of that. They were all chocolate. He couldn't wait. Terry watched anxiously as they were being handed out. Terry thought to himself, "Come on! Hurry up! Cupcakes are the best—next to doughnuts, of course."

Terry was intently watching as each one got placed in front of the other children surrounding the square, wooden tables in art class. They were big tables, and the students had to sit on stools to do their work. Finally, the teacher started handing out the cupcakes to Terry's table, and eventually his was put in front of him. He held off for just a second and decided to savor every little bit of this great moment. The fact that he didn't have his shot with him that day didn't matter. Terry was thinking of how to manage without the extra insulin. Then he noticed that the teacher stopped and said, "Wait! I almost forgot you can't have one," and picked up his cupcake. He asked her why, and she said, "I know you are not supposed to eat this because you are a diabetic." Terry looked around; everyone was staring at him. "Oh no, not now." He started to tear up, and the kid sitting on the other end of this huge, square table began making fun of him.

Joe said to Terry, "Poor baby, no cupcake for you. Do you want some of mine?" Terry said, "Sure, Joe!" Joe replied, "Psych, none for the diabetic! But you can watch me eat mine. Mmmmm, so good!" Terry said with venomous rage, "F— you!" Joe responded in kind: "Now, now, what you going to do about it? You're just a dumb diabetic!"

As Terry looked at the two kids on either side of him, who looked away, he stood up. Joe continued, "What? You going to cry now?" Terry stepped on the first rung of his stool and pushed off, sending his body to the other side of the table where Joe was sitting. Joe's cupcake just fell to the floor, and Terry smiled.

He had Joe pinned up against one of the support beams in the room. Terry's left forearm was up against his throat, and his right arm was cocked back to pound Joe's face. Terry's anger had the best of him, but he didn't care. Terry swung his arm forward toward Joe's face with his fist so tight, Terry could feel his nails digging into the palm of his hand.

Terry could sense the gazing children from all over the room, but he didn't care. He was going to get his pound of flesh. All he cared about was getting rid of all his anger, and hitting Joe was a perfect way to do just that. Terry had the drop on him. He thought, "Now is the time!"

Terry's fist came to a full stop just inches from Joe's face. The back of his arm was grabbed, and Terry was pulled off Joe. Before he could react, the teacher grabbed the hair on top of his head. Yes, the teacher actually grabbed the both of them by the hair on their heads. Talk about painful. Terry said during one of his therapy sessions, "I actually felt my feet lift off the floor." They were then escorted to the principal's office. They each told their version of the story, and Joe actually owned up to making fun of Terry. They shook hands and apologized in front of the principal. They sat in his office for the rest of the period and part of the next, when the principal finally said, "You both can go to your next class, and don't dilly dally!" Terry had home economics (he took it because he knew that lots of girls took it—and he was right), and Joe had wood shop. They walked part way back together, joking and making fun of the art teacher. Terry told Joe that they were at his class, and Joe said, "Home ec? Why?" Terry replied, "Girls!" Joe said, "Nice!" and walked on. They became best friends until his family moved away a few months later over the summer.

Home economics was boring that day, Terry said in session. "We baked some bread from scratch." Terry is actually very good at cooking and liked the class. He felt better, and he knew that the rest of the day would be great. Despite the fight, Terry had just made a new friend, and he didn't have many friends.

LUNCH PERIOD

Terry was sitting in the cafeteria, feeling a little down, and he just want to be left alone. He didn't feel like making idle chitchat with people he didn't care much about. When Terry was in the lunch line, he was still upset. He turned to an old friend for comfort and got himself a Good Humor ice cream bar. He was planning on eating it with the lunch he had brought from home. The tables were your garden-variety lunch tables with gray seats and white tops. Terry sat down at the end of one of the tables and took a deep breath. Terry took out his lunch and put the ice cream bar on the table. Before sitting, he found himself staring out the big windows as rays of light entered and illuminated the whole room. He ate by himself for most of lunch and finished his peanut butter and jelly sandwich. During one of our sessions, he recounted in his story that "I love PB&J. Mmmm!" Terry started to eat his ice cream bar. It was now soft on the inside but had a hard chocolate coating on it.

Terry hadn't noticed who was monitoring lunch until he was halfway finished with his ice cream. To his horror, Terry heard a very loud screeching voice: "Terry!!! Terry!!! McDougle!!! You get over here NOW!!!" He looked up, and on the top step of the stairs that led out to the playground was Miss B***h, the art teacher from earlier. She repeated herself: "Terry!!! Terry!!! McDougle!!! Come over here NOW!!!" Every child in seventh grade was looking at him. With his head held down, Terry walked the long journey to the steps where she waited for him.

As if Terry wasn't socially destroyed enough, she continued to dig in. Terry was halfway there and she belted out, "You are a diabetic! What are you doing eating ice cream?! You are not allowed to eat ice cream! Do you want me to call your mother? Hurry up!" Terry said that all his classmates were watching: "I then noticed several bullies staring at me, just watching, and I thought to myself, as I walked to the steps, 'I'm dead.' I realized that I had also whispered it under my breath. I then heard a classmate say, 'Yeah, you are!'"

When Terry's doctor had told him that ice cream was death on a stick, trying to scare him, he didn't think he meant being pummeled by a hoard of schoolyard bullies at recess. Terry decided he was going to skip the rest of school that day. He would just have to assure that b***h that he wouldn't do it again. He got to the art teacher but didn't recall much of the conversation. He did remember that he had forgotten to give insulin for lunch as he walked back to his table and that he didn't care. Terry threw away what was left of his ice cream, per the teacher's instructions.

The bell for recess rang. Terry grabbed his backpack and walked right out the door for recess with no intention of staying. He decided to wait until he got home to give his lunchtime insulin. Terry wasn't twenty feet away from the building when he heard, "Where do you think you're going, you diabetic pussy?" He told the kid who said that, "I don't want any problems. Just leave me alone," as he slowly set his backpack down. The bully easily had the drop on him, being at least seventy-five to one hundred pounds heavier than Terry.

Terry looked and saw the whole school watching as they piled out of the lunchroom door into the fresh air. It was still a beautiful, sunny day, and he heard someone playing Madonna's "Like a Virgin" on a boombox.

Terry was just a few feet away from the path that leads to the sport fields, which is how he walked home every day. Terry knew the drill, but still, he was thankful it was only one bully and the others were just watching. Terry was toward the bottom of a small hill. The bully had the advantage of now being at the top of the five-foot hill, standing diagonally from him. He didn't know this bully, but he looked like a dirty fighter. Terry clenched his fists as he got ready to fend off the bully's first punch. He ran toward Terry and tried to kick him. Terry jumped back, causing him to miss him by inches. The bully fell on his ass and rolled down the little hill into a puddle of water.

A split second later, Terry felt pain in his private area. The kick had landed. It was so painful that Terry struggled hard not to drop to the ground and go into a fetal position. Instead, Terry stood tall and called the bully a pussy as he stood over him. Terry grabbed his bag and started to walk away. He heard the kids in his class "laughing their asses off" behind him. Terry was happy that he was finally going home.

VICTORY SHORT LIVED

Terry was about halfway across the field. Behind him, he heard the bully yelling out, "Running away! I'm not done with you. Hey, you little shit, what's wrong? You chicken? I heard that your mother's a whore." Terry stopped in his tracks. He was standing at the end of the field, while the bully was thirty yards behind him, walking toward him. Terry didn't say

a word. He turned around and dropped his bag. He started running toward the bully, full speed with no intention of stopping. Most everyone
from his class was watching from a distance. As Terry was running, he
watched the bully stop in his tracks. Terry clenched his fists tight, and,
without stopping, he hit the bully. He watched the bully go flying back
about a good five feet and bounce off the ground. He knelt down beside
him to say, "If you ever speak to me or talk about my mother again, I
will kill you!" and then Terry walked away. He looked back and saw the
bully was still on the ground. No one was coming to help him. Terry
heard the recess bell but continued walking toward his bag. He picked
up his bag while taking one final look back. The bully was walking away
with his head held down, crying, and the other students were heading
back toward school.

Things were never the same for Terry after that day. He didn't get
into fights anymore. In fact, the school bullies would say hi as he passed
them in the halls. Terry started laughing to himself as he walked off
the field, through the back gate, on his route home. His mother wasn't
going to be there, and he wanted to be alone. During his walk home,
he noticed how sick he was feeling. By the time he got home, his blood
sugar must have been through the roof.

Terry was exhausted but glad to be home. He collapsed onto his bed
and passed out. He awoke about an hour later and started to cry. He got
up and went out onto the balcony crying. Terry found himself sitting on
the balcony handrail while thinking of leaning back and letting go. He
started to lean back, but as he started to let go, he thought to himself, "If
I do this, then that asshole bully wins." Terry's hands had already let go,
but thanks to quick reflexes and a bit of luck, he grabbed on just in time
and was now dangling nine stories up. It was a struggle for Terry, but
after a few minutes he pulled himself back over the handrail.

Still crying, with his thoughts spinning in his head, he went into his
room and laid down, relieved that he didn't fall nine stories to his death.

Terry, no longer feeling suicidal, remembered that he still hadn't
given his lunchtime insulin and checked his blood sugar. He stated

during session, "It was 426—426. I'll never forget that number or the importance of giving insulin before I eat. I hadn't thought of killing myself before that day, and I wonder how things would have gone if I had just given my shot before lunch."

A week after his suicide attempt, his mother made him go to a child psychologist for psychotherapy to help with his depression. He liked her because she helped him build skills to survive.

CHILD'S PERSPECTIVE

A child goes from feeling happy and well to nauseous and depressed inside as the day goes on and his blood sugar continues to rise. For Terry, as with many other children living with diabetes, reality gets increasingly compromised as blood sugar continues to increase. Terry had feelings of anger from previous name-calling around his diabetes. As the cupcakes were being handed out, he was simultaneously worried that he would be skipped over again and excited that maybe he wouldn't and could be like everyone else. Here is where misinformation by an un-informed teacher isolated him into social exile from his peers. Terry had feelings of loneliness around living with diabetes and his peer group. To make things worse, he felt that he had no one to talk to about these feelings because each adult Terry met made up their own rules for him, and the other kids, well, they just wouldn't understand.

Terry guessed he attacked the first kid not so much because of the name-calling as because of feeling trapped and alone with his anger—and it had to go somewhere. Even though he felt that he was in the wrong for attacking Joe, it felt good. Terry was no longer going to be this sad, pathetic little boy. He was happy that he made a new friend out of it, but at the same time, Terry was sad and down. Not even the instant gratification of an ice cream on this beautiful day perked him up. Maybe the ice cream did, for just a moment, until an unforeseen consequence occurred. Terry didn't see the consequence of eating an ice cream because it wasn't the art teacher's job to make decisions for him or implement punishment around his diabetes.

Terry had normal feelings when the teacher was screaming at him from across the room. He was mortified, embarrassed, isolated from the rest of his classmates, lonely, and scared primarily because of who was watching. He thought that he no longer cared and felt he had lost everything, so nothing mattered anymore. In session he stated, "Who cared if I had to fight every bully? I was beyond hurt. I just stopped caring at that point as I walked up to the teacher who decided it was her job to punish me. So when the bully came outside and challenged me, I wasn't scared—just numb."

Through the rest of his journey home, he was detached. When he knelt over the bully, Terry was being serious about killing him. After that point, he brought a knife into school to protect himself for a few weeks. Terry was pleased with himself after seeing the bully on the ground, but he wasn't in a good state. He was in a daze. Terry believes that his lack of concern for himself or others was the effect of the high blood sugar impacting his reality. By the time he left the bully, Terry just didn't care. He was detached and depressed. Terry stated that he didn't mean to try to kill himself on the balcony that day. He wasn't really thinking at all. Terry wondered during session, "If that teacher just hadn't singled me out. . . . Anyway, I was overwhelmed too much for one day."

PARENTAL ADVICE

This section is on the prevention of high blood sugar and the responsibility of those watching your children.

When I was growing up, there was no testing in school. In seventh grade, I never went to the nurse for anything. I carried candy to eat for low blood sugar reactions, but I never tested to see whether my blood sugar was actually low. If it felt low, I ate candy without the understanding that it could be a false reaction (blood sugar is normal but a person feels like their blood sugar is low).

Testing is critical to managing healthy blood glucose levels. It never hurts to check more often than not. If insurance is saying you can only have a certain amount of test strips, have your doctor contact the insurance and say it is medically necessary.

I test up to ten times a day if needed. In my clinical opinion, children should test or check their continuous blood glucose monitor (if they have one) before class and make adjustments as needed. If their blood sugars are in range, it will help them focus during class. If their blood sugar is high or low, depending on age and ability, they should ask for help from the teacher or nurse. Every child's needs are different. You will have to inform the school about what your child will need done for them to have a pleasant and helpful interaction with those who supervise your children while you are not there to help.

The School System

You need a plan when it comes to school. Various age groups require different levels of attention and monitoring. A big part of creating a safe environment for your child at school requires constant communication between you, the concerned parent, and the faculty at school, including the teachers, nurse, school counselor, school psychologist, and administration at all levels.

In school, there are two systems at play: the staff and your child's social network of friends and classmates. It is important to work toward helping others understand that having diabetes is normal and okay. However, keep in mind that not all children or other parents are going to believe that. It is your job to work with your child to navigate the fine balance of healthy socialization with their peers and managing the diabetes. The goal is that neither the diabetes nor your child's social network will have any significant impact on each other.

If you have followed the previous advice and downplayed the diabetes while encouraging your child to take responsibility for their actions and diabetes management when encountering other children, then this step really is a piece of cake. It is important to normalize diabetes for your child and encourage them to believe they are no different from other children, while being open to talking with them if negative feelings around their diabetes arise.

Most school systems and states have systems in place to help special needs children assimilate into school. I came across Vermont's internal program, which utilizes Legislation 504, designed to help children who are not special education but have other physical issues that need to be addressed. Vermont's 504 Legislated Program was developed by the Department of Health Diabetes Control Program (DCP). The DCP was established to reduce the impact of diabetes on children with diabetes and their families.

The Treatment Plan

There is a need to ensure your child's safety during school hours. It will be necessary to develop and implement an individualized care plan, which includes training school staff as to your child's specific needs while under their care. The treatment plan should support your child in self-care and management of their diabetes that has been recommended by their endocrinologist based on their appropriate age and abilities. It is important to include in a written treatment plan your child's physical and emotional needs and help the school understand their role in continuing the work you and your child do at home. This is necessary, as it will increase your child's opportunities to participate fully in all school activities. The treatment plan should be made in conjunction with the school and all school staff that will have daily involvement in your child's education.

The steps below are provided as a guide to the process of how your child's Individualized Care Plan is created under Legislation 504.

Step 1: Parent Conference

Make sure a parent conference is set up with those who are involved in taking care of your child at home, the principal, school nurse, and any other person you or the school feels should be at the conference. This is more of a meet-and-greet so the parties involved can get acquainted with each other and learn and share information about the school and your child. During this meeting, you will prepare for step 2 and determine who needs to be involved in step 2, "The Planning Meeting." All forms, including something similar to the one provided in appendix C, should be provided by the school prior to the parent conference.

Parent Checklist: This checklist is provided to help parents identify the forms, supplies, and other materials needed to bring to the school. The list may need to be modified based on your child's unique needs. *Some items on the checklist should be sent to the school nurse, and others your child may take with them depending on your child's age and ability to self-manage their diabetes.*

Step 2: The Planning Meeting

At the beginning of each semester, or other times of the year for children who are newly diagnosed, the school nurse should organize and facilitate the planning meeting to develop an individual diabetes care plan.

Participants may include family members, child, principal, school nurse, current year classroom teacher(s), past year classroom teacher(s),

Checklist

_____ Photograph of child
_____ Signed release of information for physician(s) (All forms are normally provided by the school)
_____ Monitoring supplies: lancets, meter, strips, alcohol, ketone strips, etc.
_____ Snack (low carb) packs. Number: _____
_____ Glucose tablets, gel (tubes). Number _____
_____ Record-keeping sheets
_____ Insulin and related supplies: syringes, alcohol, etc.
_____ Prescription medications order and permission form for insulin (All forms are normally provided by the school)
_____ Glucagon kits with premeasured dosage. Number _____
_____ Prescription medication order and permission form for glucagon (All forms are normally provided by the school)

food service manager, physical education teacher/coach, counselor or social worker, bus driver, other school staff with direct responsibility for your child, and members of the healthcare team, if invited by parents. Suggested agenda items include an overview of type 1 diabetes and its management; roles and responsibilities of staff members; identifying staff in the school who will serve as resources for others; determining the hierarchy of personnel expected to respond to emergency situations; determining the location of food kits, glucagon, and other supplies in the school building; determining where the plan will be kept and how individual components will be shared with appropriate staff; establishing how training for staff with specific responsibilities will be done; and determining what an emergency is and what to do.

Step 3: Individualized Care Plan (The School Is Responsible for Creating the ICP)

The school nurse, using information gathered at the planning meeting, needs to prepare a written plan. Key staff and the child's family must agree to the plan. The plan may be incorporated into a 504 plan if the child's needs will be covered by this legislation. All children attending public school and/or private school are partly funded under the 504 legislation.

Step 4: Training

The school nurse is responsible for arranging training for all school staff. The nurse needs to do the training with the assistance of the child's parents and/or family's healthcare team.

Online resources include Children with Diabetes (www.children-withdiabetes.com) and the American Diabetes Association (http://www.diabetes.org; http://www.diabetes.org/living-with-diabetes/parents-and-kids/diabetes-care-at-school/written-care-plans/section-504-plan.html).

I know it is a lot to take in, and a lot of work is necessary to provide proper care for your child so you won't have to worry about something similar to what happened to Terry during his education experiences in seventh and many other grades. Having a normal social life as a child is key to your child's success in life and happiness while growing up.

CLINICAL ADVICE

This section addresses blood glucose levels compared to impaired thinking and behavior.

You should watch for signs of depression, lack of motivation, spacing out, poor attention, lack of concentration, slow reaction times, and the classic frequent overactive bladder. Every individual with diabetes has a variety of these symptoms when their sugars are high or shifting from low to high.

What was happening to Terry during the course of that day in seventh grade is that his blood glucose levels rose. The ice cream was pushing it over the top. As his blood sugar increased, his emotions and ability to think clearly were impeded. This impairment is due to a lack of oxygen and increased levels of sugar in the bloodstream. High blood glucose levels hinder electrical signals in our brains that provide and receive information needed to function properly, both mentally and physically.

As this process continues, reality becomes a blur; in Terry's case, he stopped caring about the consequences of his actions. Terry couldn't have stopped the fights, but if his blood sugar had been under control, he might have gone to the principal, whom he liked and trusted, to discuss what happened at lunch.

Instead, Terry walked out—or attempted to walk out and go home. He didn't even think about the consequences. He couldn't think! It just kept getting harder and harder, as his brain was starving for oxygen. Due to the increase of sugar to the brain, his thinking was slowing because of what data could be released and received, which took longer to reach the brain, as I discussed in earlier chapters.

By the time Terry returned home, his body was shutting down and he needed to nap. Unfortunately, Terry didn't wake refreshed because his blood sugars were still high and his mind could barely understand what he was about to do. He was struggling with depression and was tired of life, and the high blood sugars fed that reality. Thank God that he had good survival instincts.

With all that said, if your child is depressed, get him/her into therapy as soon as possible. Therapy helps children cope with diabetes. Terry still attends therapy because it provides a much-needed support; it also helps to ground people who are motivated to do the work, making those who attend regularly feel better while it helps them accept and deal with their diabetes. It is a great source of support that becomes the safest place to share without the fear of being judged.

10

The Continuous Glucose Monitor Experience

WEDNESDAY, DECEMBER 2, 2015

"I don't mind that my classmates know that I have diabetes, and I don't worry or care about what they would think. After all, if they are my friends, they won't make fun of me. Some of my friends thought when I got the continuous glucose monitor (CGM) that it was cool. I spent a good part of recess showing everyone." Eric told me this in session a few months back. Now he regrets agreeing to the CGM. Eric was diagnosed in 2013 at ten years old and started working with me about a year later. He is now a very unhappy twelve-year-old.

BEFORE SCHOOL

Eric was walking to school yesterday wondering why he had been struggling to manage his blood sugars the past few weeks. He wondered whether the honeymoon period was over. Eric thought to himself, "What am I doing wrong? What is wrong with me?" Just then, his high glucose alarm went off. He ignored it, but when the second alarm rang, he sighed.

He took out his CGM and looked at it. The CGM said that he was at 220 mg/dL and rising. Eric had a big breakfast, so he didn't think there was a problem. He turned the alarm off and continued on his way to school.

He was almost at school when his phone rang. Eric didn't want to pick it up. It was his father. After the fourth ring, Eric decided to answer his phone. His father declared that he needed to test his blood sugar and give some insulin. According to what his father's phone app said, his blood sugar needed to be fixed. Some CGMs allow phone apps to receive blood glucose levels in real time via an online cloud or directly from the CGM transmitter.

Eric asked his dad if it could wait, saying, "I am only a few minutes from school. Can't it wait until I get there?" His father insisted that he check his blood sugar "now!" Eric didn't want to argue, so he tested his levels. His blood sugar was 240 mg/dL, and Eric was pleased with it. He told his dad that the number was fine because he had a big breakfast, but his father insisted that he give a correction bolus. He reluctantly agreed.

Eric was down on himself for being at 240 mg/dL, but he also felt that he shouldn't have to give a correction bolus because he had eaten breakfast an hour before and had insulin on board. However, after getting off the phone with his father, against his better judgment, he gave himself the bolus. If he didn't, his father would know.

SECOND BREAKFAST

When Eric got to school, breakfast was being served. His friends were eating, and he thought it would be good to eat with them. He enjoyed having breakfast with his friends. His best friend noticed that he did not bolus before eating. Eric told him not to worry and that he had everything under control.

Eric thought to himself, "Liar, you are such a liar!" He couldn't remember how much insulin he had given himself on the way to school or whether he had counted his carbs before eating with his friend. But he didn't have time to worry about it now, as the first period bell had just rung. He was off to class. The first period went smoothly, but he felt nauseous and very thirsty.

After class, he made a beeline to the water fountain. Then he had just enough time to go to the bathroom and his locker before the second bell rang. As he was urinating, he thought to himself that he hadn't given enough insulin for his second breakfast, so, before leaving the bathroom, he gave another bolus—and maybe a bit too much. Eric stated, "I was so confused at that point, I felt like my blood sugars were at 400 mg/dL, but I didn't know. I didn't test my blood sugar because I didn't want to be late to class."

ALWAYS LATE

Right before the second period bell rang, Eric's phone rang. His father was calling again, and he was forced to check his blood glucose and be late to class. Now he was unintentionally compelled to sneak into class late. To his dismay, the door slammed shut behind him and everyone stared.

The teacher was upset and said, "Mr. Smith, you seem to not understand what the second bell means. So, what is your excuse this time? Well, Mr. Smith? I'm waiting!" Eric looked down and said, "Uuuuh, I don't know." The teacher told him to go ahead and take his seat and stated, "You are not in kindergarten anymore. Please act like it and be in your seat when the bell rings!" He sat down and noticed that some students were still looking at him. He took out his book as the teacher started her lesson. Eric made it through the rest of the second period without incident, and art class was next.

ART CLASS

His anxiety was drifting away because his art teacher knew he had diabetes and understood his situation. It was also his best subject. Eric stepped into the art class and noticed that there was a substitute teacher, but he was still happy to be there, even if they weren't going to be learning anything new.

Eric's class was drawing a still life of everyday objects that his favorite teacher had left for them. Halfway through class, his phone rang. He went for the button to silence it; then he answered the phone and whispered, "Yes, okay, okay, three glucose tabs. All right, will do."

PHONE POLICY AT SCHOOL

Eric was embarrassed, despite the fact that he was given permission to use his phone in school. His school had a strict no-phone policy. If that wasn't bad enough, the substitute was staring right at him and told him to turn off the phone. However, Eric couldn't turn it off, or he would have gotten in trouble at home. He tried to explain that he was allowed to have it on, but the teacher wouldn't hear it and sent him to the principal's office.

He started to tear up as he grabbed his backpack and began his journey to the principal's office. As he opened the classroom door, one of the school's bullies said, "About time! Have fun with the principal!" Two or three of the other children he didn't know chimed in and said, "Yeah! Have fun," and then laughed. As Eric walked down the hallway, he started crying. Part of him knew he was not going to get in trouble, but another part didn't believe it.

This was not his first time at the principal's office, but it felt like it. Eric was still crying as he entered the office. Expecting the worst, he looked up at the principal. The principal asked what had happened, and Eric told him. The principal was a tall, stocky man who struck fear into even the worst kids in school, but he kneeled down and gave Eric a big hug and, in a warm, soft voice, said, "Everything is going to be okay. It was just a misunderstanding." Eric didn't want to face the kids in class, and it seemed his principal knew it.

He spent the rest of the period talking with the principal. He was grateful for the pleasant talk and the time to recoup. The bell rang, and he went off to class. No more than a minute after sitting down—you guessed it—his phone rang. He told his father to hold on. Eric went to his teacher and asked whether he could step into the hallway. His teacher said okay and gave him the hall pass.

In a stressed voice, his father asked whether he had checked his blood sugar and eaten the three glucose tablets like he said. Eric said, "No, but . . ." "I don't want to hear it! You know better! What are you doing? You are in so much trouble!" "But it wasn't my fault." His father said, "I don't want to hear it! Just check your blood sugar."

Eric checked it—55 mg/dL. "Well, what is it?!" "55." "What? Are you just ignoring your alarms on your CGM?" "No, I am not." "Well, we will deal with this when you get home! For now, take four glucose tablets, and I expect you to call me back in fifteen minutes with test results, or you're grounded."

Eric took the four glucose tablets, realized he had forgotten to turn his CGM alarms back on, and proceeded to fix that. He then set an alarm on his phone to go off in fifteen minutes. It went off as planned. He checked his blood sugar, which was now at 84. He called his father, told him the results, and went back to class.

LUNCHTIME

During lunch, Eric was visibly upset. His friends asked him what was wrong. He told them not to worry about it. After all, what had happened that morning was not abnormal for Eric. It was just another day dealing with diabetes—since starting on the CGM, anyway. Eric checked his blood sugar before eating. It was at 187 mg/dL. Not wanting another call from his dad, he decided to think out his next decision carefully. It was a risky one but on the money.

Eric gave a correction bolus and a bolus to cover lunch, since he knew that he had no insulin on board and that it would take a while for his bolus to work. He ate half his sandwich and left the other half of his sandwich, plus his potato chips, to eat at recess. He went ahead and set his alarm for forty-five minutes as a reminder. At recess, his blood sugar had started to go down, and Eric ate the rest of his lunch. He stated, "I avoided the slingshot effect [the Somogyi effect, also known as the rebound effect]. I was in range the rest of the day, but I still had another call from my dad during seventh period. I was ready for it."

Between sixth and seventh periods, Eric was alerted to a high blood sugar that seemed off to him. The CGM was stating that his blood sugar was 203 mg/dL, but when he tested his blood sugar, it was actually at 130 mg/dL and well within range. He tested again and saw that his glucose level was 125 mg/dL. He recalibrated his CGM, and everything was fine—or so he thought, anyway.

It wasn't but five minutes into class when his father called. He had done this many other times when Eric's CGM needed recalibration. Due to a delay from the CGM to the cloud, and from the cloud to his father's phone, his father would react to old information. Eric answered the phone. Before his father could speak, he told him that his blood sugar was fine and he had recalibrated the CGM. There was a pause. When his father finally spoke, he said, "Okay, but you are still in trouble." He also told Eric that he had told his therapist all about what had happened that day.

At the beginning of our next session, I told Eric that I had received a call from his dad. I assured Eric that diabetes is difficult for everyone, including parents. I said, "We can discuss what happened between you and your father in our upcoming family session. Today's meeting is for you, and if you want to talk about yesterday, it's your choice. From what your father said, I am sure it was a rough day for you."

Eric responded, "I get that my parents are scared that something bad is going to happen to me. I realize that! But ever since getting the CGM, my parents just won't leave me alone."

CHILD'S PERSPECTIVE

Eric had been looking forward to going on the CGM for weeks prior to its arrival. He felt that the CGM would reduce the number of times he would have to test his blood sugar. When he finally received his CGM, he was so excited. Eric felt that going on the CGM would also cause his father to calm down and he could relax a bit. Eric thought it would reduce the number of diabetes-related discussions. He was hoping it would make things a bit easier on him and his worries.

Before getting diabetes, Eric was a responsible child with good grades in school. He had lots of friends and participated in several after-school activities. He didn't mind that his classmates knew because after being diagnosed with diabetes, he had already lost some friends due to misunderstandings around his diabetes. However, because of all of his accomplishments, he originally felt a sense of security when it came to managing the day-to-day tasks of living with diabetes.

Weight of the World

Even though Eric stated that he didn't mind that his classmates knew about diabetes, it was because the handful of friends who stuck around were already supportive. He did care about what his friends would think. After much discussion, over several therapy sessions, he came to recognize his denial and that he was afraid of losing more friends and ending up all alone.

Before diabetes, Eric didn't worry about much, except getting good grades or making the basketball team. After being diagnosed, he worried about things like diabetes self-management and the difficulties that come with it, like high blood sugar and low blood sugar, as well as death and dying, for example.

He was also concerned about being punished for having diabetes. Diabetes complications and knowing where the nearest bathroom is at all times were on his mind as well. Eric was fearful about being singled out as different by adults and teachers, losing friends, and being noticed by the school bullies. Eric was always stressed about how his classmates would see him, angering his parents, pleasing his parents, and being a burden on his family and friends.

Eric blamed himself for everything that happened to him, as many children do, such as when a young child overhears parents arguing. Most young children instantly believe it is about them, when in reality chances are that it doesn't have anything to do with the children.

His illness, his fault—and, in Eric's case, this idea was supported by his father's blame and anger. He heard things like "You used to be so responsible. Why didn't you do . . . [this or that]? You should know better by now." Eric's father would say, "If you took better care of your diabetes, we wouldn't have to . . ." Eric was confused since he was doing the best he could. In the past, he would receive praise and lots of "Atta boy! Great job!" comments from his father. He was still doing his best, but now he got lots of guilt and blame. "After all, how could it be anyone else's fault but mine?" Eric stated in one of our first sessions together.

Over the past year, he has come to realize it isn't his fault, because diabetes just happens, and he can't control everything. Eric knows this logically, but his emotional self still makes him think otherwise, especially when people around him or cognitive distortions of high blood glucose support that feeling. It was one of those days. Eric's logical mind was not available due to the cognitive impact of high blood sugars. It is difficult for adults to make good judgment calls when blood sugar is high, but the younger you are, the worse it is.

Eric was already feeling sad and blaming himself for not doing what he felt he should be doing to keep his blood sugar in range. A lot of children living with diabetes, even children much younger than Eric, may feel that way but may not be able to express it because of age, the inability to understand their feelings, or the fact that the environment at home doesn't encourage or support emotional expression.

Eric felt like his opinion didn't matter and was unsure in his decisions around management. It is important to remember your child's age. Eric is nowhere close to an adult despite acting like it sometimes; yet his parents believed that he should be taking care of his diabetes like an adult.

Taking into account that the majority of adults living with diabetes struggle with diabetes management and the emotions that come with it every day, it is important to remember that children living with diabetes have to manage the same issues. The younger a child is, the more confusing everything becomes.

Eric was right about the honeymoon period ending and the need to change his insulin regimen, but his uncertainty, self-blame, and self-doubt caused him to overlook that and spiral into self-shaming. Always afraid of his father's negative attention, he struggles to pick up the phone. He eventually answers the phone because the repercussions of not picking it up would upset his father, and he might have to deal with his mother's anger as well.

However, the consequence of picking up the phone was worse. His heightened anxiety and fear caused Eric to doubt himself. If his father had been willing to listen to him during that first call, and if Eric had been in a position to advocate for himself, then things might have gone differently that day. I say this because Eric was correct about waiting for the blood sugars to go down on their own.

While happy about meeting his friends for breakfast in the cafeteria, he was also worried about the extra insulin. Even though his friends knew he has diabetes, he still doesn't want to put it front and center. He knew better but felt social pressure and started eating without figuring out the carbs to know whether he needed to give more for the extra food, even though, at this point, it would have been tough to calculate due to insulin stacking as well as Eric's impaired memory, logic, and judgment caused by his high blood sugar. It is similar to that cloudy, foggy, unclear, and woozy part of a head cold where you can't think straight.

Between a Rock and Hard Place

Issues like choosing between being on time to class and taking care of the diabetes is a common occurrence for children in school. Children with diabetes have many conflicting responsibilities. As Eric goes through his day, he has to balance these responsibilities: social, education, family, and health.

The healthy choice is not always put first, but if you are a twelve-year-old trying to balance an immense amount of responsibilities, the choice seems clear. Either you are a social outcast for the next few years or you feel sick for a few extra hours of high blood sugar. Although not logical, many adults with diabetes would also pick having a few extra hours of bad blood glucose over not fitting in at work.

Most likely, your child with diabetes feels angry, frustrated, sad, scared, and confused about the choices they have to make on a daily basis.

Think back to your childhood. Remember how everything changed when you were starting your teen years, when wearing the wrong type of shoe was uncool, how important it was to fit into your respective group, and when being different was not a good thing.

Children with diabetes are more likely to be bullied because they are different, and getting extra attention at school, even unwanted attention, is a bad thing—like when the smartest kid in your class gets extra attention from the teacher. Other classmates might call them a nerd or stuck-up because they are angry that they aren't getting extra attention, whether they deserve it or not.

Since children living with diabetes look like everyone else, most children would look at Eric being able to answer his phone or text in class as a privilege. Being different can make you a social outcast, so many kids hide their diabetes to fit in and will sacrifice good management to be socially accepted in school and even at home.

PARENTAL ADVICE

Think back to your childhood. Remember how complicated life was, and ask yourself whether you could have made life-and-death choices on a daily basis. At what age did you understand the concept of life and death? For most people, it takes a lifetime to understand the concept of life and death. Now imagine how overwhelming it must be for your child.

I know it is scary for you too. It is normal to be concerned about the safety of one's child as a parent, up to a point. Too much concern becomes worry, and you start doing things like Eric's father, spending hours on end looking at his phone, losing sleep, and sacrificing his job while unintentionally having an adverse impact on his family.

Diabetes is a family illness and affects all members of the family, and, as such, all family members may need emotional help, professional support from a certified diabetes educator (CDE), and continued education throughout the developmental period of your child's life.

Eric's father was scared and overly reactive. Therefore, he missed that it had only been an hour since breakfast. Fear and the need to control are a dangerous combination when raising a child living with diabetes. I know some of you reading this are saying, "What? Are you out of your gourd? How can I not fear this illness? Don't we need to control diabetes?"

Some Fear

Some amount of fear is necessary, but too much can cause a parent to become overprotective, suffocating their child's independence. A parent might treat their twelve-year-old as though he or she is five years old. Every perceived management mistake can cause a parent to trust their child less and less. For example, when Eric turned off his CGM's alarm or forgot to turn it back on, it can be seen as a mistake, lack of care, or deliberate. Various perceived management mistakes caused Eric's father to stop trusting him. Believe it or not, most children and adolescents want to take care of their diabetes and care about their health, and their behaviors are not deliberate.

Unfortunately, this misperception around management accidents happens to a lot of parents. As time goes on, the child, out of a need for independence and fear of punishment, will stop sharing relevant management information, pulling the child and parent further and further apart and increasing fear levels exponentially.

Children need to feel that they can talk about what they are going through without judgment. It is important to remember that no matter how responsible they act, they are still children. It is also critical to provide age-appropriate parenting.

Regardless of the problem they are facing with their diabetes or school, they need to know that they are not alone and you will work with them as part of their team to resolve the issues that happen. They need to know that you will listen to them and that they are heard in a nonbiased and nonjudgmental environment.

In Eric's situation, the CGM catalyzed his father's fear that diabetes will kill his son. For some, this is an unfortunate consequence of getting the CGM for their child, but it can be remedied by talking with a CDE or a psychotherapist to help parents manage their expectations and the intense emotions caused by diabetes, such as fear, frustration, sadness, or guilt. It is extra hard to raise a child with diabetes, but having someone to talk to can help.

I believe that information is a good thing, but too much information is overwhelming, like knowing your child's blood sugar every moment of every day, as in Eric's case. This situation is where having the cloud feature could be unnecessarily stressful. It left Eric's father feeling powerless to help his son and contributed to his intense need to control.

Management

Many parents feel they need to control everything for their children to be safe, which could not be further from the truth. It is impossible to control every aspect of your child's life without diabetes in the picture. Diabetes also can't be controlled, but it can be managed. If you feel that you can control it or make attempts to control it, you will always come up short.

The best we can hope to do is manage it. So why do we think we need to or can control something as complicated as diabetes? When we believe we can control everything, it creates a feeling of safety and security, although not based in reality. In the end, we can only control our actions—and not even that all the time. Very few people can buy a pint of ice cream or a bag of potato chips and eat just one serving at a time. It is part of being human.

In some areas of diabetes, management can be controlled. We can count carbs and give the proper amount of insulin, but if our metabolism is a little higher than the previous day, our blood sugar may go low anyway. We can control having glucose nearby when low blood sugar happens. If your child is going through puberty, their hormones are all over the place, and even though the appropriate amount of insulin has been given, it may not be enough because hormone levels increased and most hormones besides insulin raise glucose levels.

At the end of Eric's day, he stated that he was trying to control for the Somogyi effect. The Somogyi effect, also known as the "rebound" effect, was named after Michael Somogyi, who first recognized it. After blood glucose levels drop low, the body may release counter regulatory hormones such as glucagon and epinephrine. If your body produces insulin, then that is not an issue, but for someone with diabetes, it can be very taxing. This is one of the unpredictable aspects of management.

So it is important to change your views around control. Accepting that diabetes can't be controlled and that it is tough to manage may help you accept that it is okay when your child's blood sugar goes high or low. The best anyone, including myself, can hope to do is manage diabetes the best we can, and the CGM helps us do that.

Starting the CGM

Depending on the age of your child, they might have an issue with going on a CGM. For some kids, it won't be a problem at all, but a lot of children experience emotional turmoil for various reasons. Some may not want to be continuously reminded that they are different, that they have diabetes. Others may have issues related to body image and fitting in with the other children in school.

One thing is for sure: they need to be part of the decision process. Children need to feel that it is their choice to go on the CGM. Without it, you will be stuck with an uphill battle.

If your child is not part of the decision-making process, they may decide that they don't want any part of the CGM and start acting out.

Some children who don't want to be on the CGM might be passive about it at first. After telling your child that they are going on the CGM, they may or may not ask questions about the CGM, but, questions or not, they will tell you what you want to hear. You believe they are on board, but deep down they may be resentful that they have to do more work to take care of their diabetes.

After the CGM arrives, they may be resistant to using it. When your child is on their own, they might do things to impede or prevent the CGM from working. A thirteen-year-old client of mine would tell her parents that her transmitter kept falling off. Her parents paid for many replacement transmitters.

During our session, she said that she deliberately removed the transmitters, figuring that her parents would eventually give up and take her off the CGM. She stated that they never asked whether she wanted to use a CGM. She also said, "I wish they had asked me before getting it. I hate the color. Just because I am a girl doesn't mean I want or like the color pink. Nothing I say matters. This is just another way for my parents to control me."

Another client of mine, nineteen years old and living at college, would not put the transmitter on until his parents called. At the same time, he would not enter blood sugar levels into the receiver, which is needed for the CGM to calibrate or work properly.

Children need to feel that they have a say in the matter and have some control over how to manage their diabetes. It is important that they are part of the decision-making process so they will be motivated to implement changes in management.

It is important to allow them to make age-appropriate decisions around all aspects of managing their diabetes. For the very young, getting to pick the color of the CGM will have a profound impact on their desire and motivation to follow parental instructions around diabetes management. Making diabetes a team effort can help your child feel supported instead of isolated.

At a certain point, it is important for children growing up with diabetes to take over managing their diabetes. A slow transition period in the early teen years will give them confidence and allow you to trust that they will manage their diabetes when you are not around.

Where It Helps

The CGM is designed to help you and your son or daughter (age dependent) make better management choices and warns of low and high blood sugar, so you can react faster to out-of-range blood glucose levels.

For many parents, the CGM is a godsend. For young children, there are baby monitor CGMs that will sound an alarm in the parent's bedroom when blood sugars are out of range, allowing the parents to have a restful sleep, knowing they will be woken up when blood sugar drops below or above a certain level. For older children, any number of CGMs will wake them up to address low and high blood sugar.

The CGM is great. It helps with better management and increases the user's safety and their feeling of security. Remember, nothing with diabetes runs smoothly, especially in the beginning. If your child forgets to check their blood sugar before eating once in a while, that is normal. Adults living with diabetes go through the same things: forgetting to turn their CGM alarm back on, forgetting to check blood sugar, or forgetting insulin once in a while is normal. When it becomes a daily issue, there is some underlying problem that needs to be addressed. If your child does forget insulin, the CGM will help them realize it.

CLINICAL ADVICE

This section is on choosing the best CGM for your child and working with your healthcare team.

CGMs make a big difference in the ability to manage blood sugar level, create a feeling of safety, and reduce fear around low blood sugars, while decreasing your child's HbA1c results.

The data collected helps detect patterns in blood sugar levels over the course of weeks, allowing people of all ages living with diabetes and their doctors make better-informed decisions around changes in management.

There are many things to think about when picking a CGM, and yes, color choice is one of them. Not all CGMs come in different colors. Color may not be your primary concern. Whether your endocrinologist recommends or has the necessary tool to download and evaluate the data may be your biggest concern. All options available should be taken into account when buying a CGM.

If you have lived with and actively managed your diabetes for twenty years, you may choose the most accurate CGM on the market, even if your endocrinologist recommends a different monitor. The decision needs to meet your needs and be personalized for your unique circumstance. (I want to make a note here that infants to teenagers can wear a CGM, and it can bring peace of mind for the parents. Just keep in mind Eric's father's experience and recognize that there is a delay with all CGMs and checking blood sugar is important for correction doses as well as for verifying low blood sugars.)

Some Unique Monitor Options

Some CGM receivers are incorporated into certain pumps. This kind of pump allows the user to carry one less piece of equipment around with them. It may or may not be part of a closed system pump where the CGM instructs the pump to add or reduce insulin.

At one point, there was a baby monitor/receiver, but I believe it has been taken off the market. Fortunately, the FDA has approved some CGMs for children ages two to seventeen, while some CGMs have a range of twenty feet, allowing parents to put the receiver by their bed and not have to keep checking in on their child throughout the night.

Medical Consultation

It is important to consult with your endocrinologist or certified diabetes educator when choosing what CGM to purchase. Several things need to happen before getting your CGM. Most health insurances require three months of documented blood sugars along with a prescription from your endocrinologist.

Once your healthcare team helps you decide on a CGM that is most appropriate for your child, you may need to contact your health insurance company. Some healthcare providers or medical suppliers may

Table 10.1. CGM Options

Color	What colors does it come in?
Screen	How big is the screen? Can I clearly read it? Is it backlit so I can read in the dark? Monochrome or color?
Display	Is it a touch screen display?
Transmitter/Sensor Size	How small and noticeable is it to others?
Sensor Life	How long until I have to change the sensor? They presently range from three to ten days before requiring replacement.
The Angle of Insertion	Discuss with your endocrinologist what angle will work best with your body type if needed.
Insertion Device	Does it have an insertion device, or is it manual insertion? (An insertion device automatically injects the sensor into the body. Most CGMs have one that comes in the box.)
Initialization Time	How long will you have to wait after the sensor is injected before you can start using the monitor?
Alarms	How adjustable are they? Can you set the alarms for different times throughout the day and night, different sounds for each alarm, and how loud the alarms are?
Predictive Alarms	Is there an alarm that can be set to warn before the glucose limit has been reached?
The Rate of Change	Does the CGM have an alarm that can warn when blood sugar is rising or falling too quickly?
Glucose Data	Where can you review it? Phone, receiver, online?
Review Glucose Data	How can you interpret glucose data and length of time (i.e., twenty-four hours, one week, one month, etc.)?
Record Events	Do you have the ability to enter insulin, exercise, carbs, or other health data?
Alarm Types	Can it vibrate or/and escalate (sound increases) when low or high blood glucose isn't attended to?
Waterproof	Is the transmitter or receiver waterproof?
Batteries	What type of battery is needed, and is it rechargeable? How long does the charge last?
Range	What is the maximum distance the receiver can be from the transmitter and still record data?
Computer Software	Does it work on both PC and Mac?
Upgrade	Is there a program in place that allows you to upgrade when a newer model comes on the market?
Customer Service	Does the CGM company have a good track record?

contact your insurance on your behalf to obtain the necessary documentation and see what CGMs are covered.

This process may go smoothly, or you may have to fight to get the CGM, so be prepared. If your doctor prescribes a CGM, it means that the device is medically necessary. Some insurance companies will approve only certain CGM brands, but they can't deny it altogether. They may try to deny based on the blood sugar results from the collected blood glucose diary you provided the insurance company. In that case, your doctor might have to go to bat for you and contact your insurance company.

Regardless of whether everything goes smoothly, it is worth fighting for, so don't give up trying, and be an advocate for your child. Insurance companies like saying no, but you can escalate all the way to the CEO. I have seen insurance companies change their decision. Good luck.

11

The Insulin Pump Process

SATURDAY, DECEMBER 13, 2008

Tom was excited! It was his thirteenth birthday, and his parents had promised him that when he turned thirteen years old, he could get a pump. Tom asked his parents, "So, it's my birthday, and you know what that means?" His mother paused for a moment and said, "I'm sorry, Tom. We talked to the doctor, and he stated that it wasn't medically necessary, plus the insurance won't cover it. I discussed it with your father, and we can't afford to pay for it ourselves. We are very sorry, Tom." His dad jumped in and said, "Tom, I know you are disappointed, but, unfortunately, it is out of our control. We did get you some great presents for your birthday."

THE STANDOFF

Tom recalls just looking at the floor after he heard the bad news. He looked up to his father's glare for what seemed like forever. Tom searched for words, but none came to mind as he slowly looked away from his parents. He put his jacket on without a word; then he walked out the door. He thought to himself, "I just can't deal with this!"

Upon returning home, he told his parents he was fine: "Don't worry. If diabetes has taught me anything, it is not to get your hopes up."

"Don't say that," his mother said. He looked at the ground and went into his room.

He thought to himself how none of his friends had to deal with this kind of stuff, and how excited his friends would be at getting a new computer for their birthdays, but Tom wasn't. Tom thought that he was not like the other kids at school. He had diabetes, and he kept getting reminded of it.

Tom didn't want his parents to let this go. He had ongoing conversations with them over the next six months. Tom was pragmatic about the situation. In these talks with his parents, he pointed out every piece of research he could find that led to better control with the pump. His parents kept insisting that his endocrinologist said the insurance wouldn't cover it and that his HbA1c didn't need improvement.

His parents were getting frustrated and did not budge from their stance on the pump. Tom even said he would get a job to help pay for it. No dice. Eventually his parents told him that they would bring it up with his endocrinologist at their next appointment, but there was a catch: if the endocrinologist said no after they made a case for it, Tom would have to let it go.

ENDOCRINOLOGIST'S OFFICE

Tom and his parents were sitting in the waiting room at his endocrinologist's office. Tom thought that he would present his research and the doctor would see that it was medically necessary. Tom was sure of it! He thought that his doctor would be open to his perspective and the research he had found to back it up.

Once again, he was going to be his usual pragmatic self. Certainly his doctor would see his point of view. After all, it was research based, his numbers were good, and he had always been a responsible kid. Tom thought that being responsible meant the doctor would see that he would take good care of the pump and follow the rules, and that being responsible could sway his doctor into telling the insurance company that he was ready for the pump.

Tom heard his name called. He was very excited, popped up out of the waiting room chair, and practically ran to the nurse, with his parents following closely behind him. The nurse took him to the second waiting room. He always hated the second waiting room because it felt like being tricked. After what seemed like forever, the doctor came in.

The doctor commended him on his excellent management and how happy he was with his HbA1c. Tom couldn't recall what it was back then but knew it was better than most people his age—according to the doctor, anyway.

The doctor wouldn't budge on his decision and reiterated what he had told Tom's parents. Tom said, "It is like you are punishing me for managing my diabetes well." His doctor didn't know what to say except "There would be little difference in your HbA1c, so it is not necessary." Tom replied in anger, "Maybe I should stop managing my diabetes so well then!"

Tom didn't talk much on the ride home. His parents said they were sorry, and he responded like most teenagers would: "Whatever!" Tom was upset that his parents didn't step in, didn't say a word in the doctor's office or make an effort to help him convince the doctor that the pump would be a good thing to have.

They got home, and Tom thought about what the doctor said. He understood his point but felt anything that would improve his management would be a good thing to have. What the doctor said didn't change the fact that a pump would improve his already good numbers, or that he was still angry at his parents, or that he still felt it was important to get an insulin pump.

ONE YEAR LATER

At school, he met another teen his age living with diabetes who already had the pump. He asked him all sorts of questions and discovered something interesting. Tom was now armed and ready to bring the pump up again with his doctor.

D-DAY: DECEMBER 21, 2010

It has been more than two years since his first discussion with his parents about going on a pump. Tom was now fifteen years old and more attuned to the ways of the world. He felt even more confident that he was going to change his doctor's mind.

He waited patiently for the door to open and the doctor to enter the other waiting room. It seemed like forever, but Tom said it was probably only five minutes. The doctor arrived and said, "Well, Tom, another great HbA1c, and everything else looks great. I wish my other teens had your numbers." Tom responded, "That's great, but the numbers could be better with a pump." The doctor's face got stern, and once again he said that his HbA1c was too good for the pump to be medically necessary.

Tom thought he had him right where he wanted him: "I heard from a friend of mine that if the insurance company says it is not medically necessary, you could intervene on my behalf like my friend's doctor did for him." The doctor's response was dismissive.

The doctor talked about each patient being unique and on and on. Eventually, the speech was over. Tom knew that he had lost this battle, but the war was still on. He was now even more determined.

On the ride home, he kept thinking about his doctor's long-winded speech and each point he made. He found one of his doctor's statements where he was labeled as a typical adolescent particularly offensive. "How dare he say that about me?" he thought to himself. "I am not like every other teenager." The doctor's statement was "In my experience and medical observations, teenagers don't do well on the pump and, if anything, their HbA1c goes up."

TOM'S MULTIPLE ATTEMPTS

Tom tried many approaches over the next three years. He had many conversations with his parents. They believed that it was impossible to buy the pump out of pocket or get the pump through insurance. He had many conversations with his friends, and while they had some interesting ideas, like stealing a pump or buying a gun and forcing the doctor to change his mind, they were far from helpful.

At the doctor's office, all he heard was "not medically necessary." Not medically necessary, over and over again. He couldn't figure it out until one day, while sitting in class, it came to him.

At his next appointment, Tom said to his endocrinologist, "You know, the HbA1c only tells part of the story, doesn't it?" The doctor appeared to be listening, just as Tom had listened attentively during a recent statistics class. He said to the physician, "Do you realize that there is a difference between a median, a mode, and a mean?" The doctor replied, "Yes, but what does this have to do with diabetes?"

Tom replied, "I will tell you. I was sitting in math class, bored out of my mind, while the teacher was explaining the difference between the median, mode, and mean. All that changed when he started to explain the mean. At that point I realized that the HbA1c is a mean. The teacher said, 'A mean is the average of an entire set of numbers,' just like the HbA1c.

"My math teacher said, 'The downside is that it doesn't tell you the whole story. It doesn't show you the highest number or the lowest number or how far apart the numbers are and all the numbers in between.' How do you know when looking at a patient's HbA1c that his or her blood sugars are stable and in range the majority of the time?"

The doctor said that he didn't know. Tom then asked, "How do you know whether I am in good control?" The doctor replied, "I don't really know. I just assumed that you would tell me if your blood sugars were all over the place."

Tom told the doctor, "Well, Doc, you thought wrong. My daily blood sugars are far from perfect, and since my parents didn't come this time and aren't sitting next to me, I can tell you the truth." Tom's doctor was visibly upset by this news. By the end of the appointment, his doctor requested that Tom journal his blood sugars and gave him a form. He told Tom that "if this is true," he might need to be on the pump after all.

Two weeks later, Tom gave the doctor his journal. The doctor saw that his blood sugars were not stable and requested that he write down all of his blood sugars over the next three months. Tom said, "Three months! That seems a bit excessive." His doctor told him that the insurance would need that information to approve the pump, and then the doctor exited the room.

VICTORY! (ALMOST)
Tom sat there for a few minutes with a smile on his face—more like a grin. He had finally won. He still had to make sure the numbers were off enough to be medically necessary, just like he had done for the past two weeks.

Tom said to himself that he would figure out fixing the numbers over the next three months. After all, Tom was in good control, but he knew it could be better, even if the insurance company didn't agree.

Tom also stated that he wished he had thought of his plan sooner, but he didn't have a statistics class until twelfth grade. Based on Tom's report, he was doing great for a high school student living with diabetes.

He decided to inflate the numbers as he was journaling, just like he did for his first journal. The number 180 mg/dL he would change to a number above 200 mg/dL, 80s became 60s, and so on. Some days he just made it up. When done, he felt sure that he had hit it out of the park. He met with his endocrinologist a month before his eighteenth birthday, which was the day he got the news that his insurance had approved his pump.

The best part was that six months later, his HbA1c dropped from 7.0 to 6.4 with increased blood sugar stability. Tom was in the best control of his life.

CHILD'S PERSPECTIVE
Tom had been looking forward to going on the pump for several months before his thirteenth birthday. He believed that the pump would reduce the number of carb/insulin ratio mistakes he was having and prevent him from stacking his insulin. When Tom discovered that he could not get a pump as expected, he was disappointed, angry, sad,

frustrated, and confused. He felt he deserved the pump, and he wasn't going to let anyone say otherwise.

His parents said that it wasn't their choice; it was the doctor's. For Tom, that made the situation even worse, causing feelings of resentment and anger toward his parents. He felt that they didn't put up a fight or advocate for him.

Even though most teenagers might say they don't want their parents involved in their lives, teens do want some involvement. After all, being an adolescent is about testing one's independence, not being 100 percent independent, while having a safe place to retreat to when things get tough. It is similar for teenagers living with diabetes, but managing this disorder may confuse them or make them less adventurous when it comes to pushing the boundaries of their independence and the need for parental support.

Tom needed his parents to be supportive at that moment but was confused because he was taught to follow the doctor's advice, even though he knew the doctor was wrong. He also believed his parents knew it but did nothing. Regardless of not knowing what his parents did or didn't do or why his doctor felt it wasn't medically necessary, Tom felt he knew best.

Tom's pragmatic approach was sound but flawed, as medical necessity doesn't have much to do with prevention. The more conversations and resistance on his parents' part, the more angry and frustrated he got. His anger propelled him forward to prove the doctor wrong. Tom's frustration over the resistance he got from the doctor, insurance company, and his parents caused him to feel all alone and made him want to curl up into a ball and die.

Tom went on his walk after being told that he wasn't going to get a pump. He decided that he was going to fight this. He felt like he was taking on the world but hoped that he could get people to listen to him.

Tom tried to get his parents to see that the doctor was wrong and that it was medically necessary. After each attempt, he felt angry, sad, and lonely. He couldn't understand why his parents didn't care about his health, even though they did very much. Many times when children get angry, they forget about the good things their parents have done for them.

Eventually, his parents caved and said that they would bring it up with the doctor, but he didn't trust them. After hearing the doctor say that it wasn't medically necessary, he was still angry and sad, as well as hopeless. While his parents thought it was over, he became even more driven.

Tom felt it was unfair that other children living with diabetes could get the pump and he had to fight for it. Despite the support of his friend who had diabetes and the support of his other friends, he felt alone with his illness. Every time he had a new approach, he got excited and hopeful. After each time he talked to his doctor and he refused to help, Tom stopped believing in his doctor and stopped following his suggestions. After his latest approach had failed, he became angry with himself for not getting the pump. He was disappointed that no one was helping him.

As time went on, Tom became more and more detached. He didn't care about getting the pump toward the end. He was exhausted and burned out. He had all but given up when that fateful day came and he started to understand what the HbA1c showed. He became excited again but wasn't going to get his hopes up.

When the doctor said that he would submit to the insurance, Tom was worried but excited. He felt vindicated but believed that he needed to misrepresent his blood sugar levels to make sure he got the pump. He felt guilty about lying but also felt that he did the right thing. His health was more important than feeling a little guilt. He was right; the more controlled a person living with diabetes is at the time they fill out the blood sugar diary, the less likely it is that insurance will pay for it.

After getting the pump, he started worrying about what his friends would think. His friends knew, but Tom was worried that if he put diabetes management up front, he might lose his friends. He thought about hiding it but chose not to, and his friends came through for him.

They continued to be supportive by asking a few questions. When he told them that he didn't want to talk about his diabetes anymore, they backed off.

Life for Tom went on as it did in the past. Nothing much changed, except that he felt better physically and emotionally. Tom said that some days when his blood sugars were in range and stable, he felt normal. This excited Tom because he had never felt this healthy before, and he was ecstatic when he saw his blood sugar levels improve.

PARENTAL ADVICE

In my mind, the pump will always be about prevention and therefore medically necessary. When dealing with various doctors and nurses, decisions around your child's health can be made easier or more complicated. In Tom's case, his doctor made it more difficult than it needed to be.

His endocrinologist could have taken a different approach. While it might seem that he wouldn't get approved for the pump, the doctor doesn't know until the patient actually tries. Some doctors advocate and go that extra mile for their patient, but Tom's doctor didn't.

What the doctor can do is sometimes different from what they actually do. Let's say Tom's doctor agreed with Tom and the insurance company said no. His doctor, as well as his parents, could have made an appeal.

Advocating for your child is important. In this case, Tom's parents could have advocated for the physician to submit the paperwork the insurance company needs to see whether they approve it or get a second opinion. Once you find an endocrinologist willing to prescribe a pump, they may help you get it by filling out the necessary paperwork and submitting it to the insurance company for you.

His parents could have contacted the insurance company directly and asked them what their process is around getting a pump. Some insulin pump companies have customer service representatives that can help in this process and may even contact the insurance company for you. There are also intermediaries (third-party supply companies) that can help patients with the process, provided you use their services.

If you don't ask what your options are, then you are stuck with the medical community's and the insurance company's answer.

Encouragement and Support

Without the backing of his parents or a certified diabetes educator like me, Tom would still manage to succeed despite taking much longer than needed. After five years of trying different approaches, Tom did succeed. He didn't have the knowledge to get a second opinion or escalate his approach like his parents could. He is an example for every parent out there who has to deal with a doctor not willing to go the extra mile or the insurance company saying no.

I had a parent who escalated all the way to the CEO of their insurance company and got reimbursed for my services. Just think how much better Tom's life would have been if his parents had gotten that second opinion. It might have been a struggle, but I know it would have taken less time and Tom would not have spent five years of his life feeling angry, sad, or lonely about getting a pump.

There are many roadblocks to getting medical equipment like a pump. Everyone's experience with the medical community and insurance companies is different. Some are helpful, but many are not. You have to learn what your insurance plan provides and reach out to the various entities that can help you. If you are told no by the insurance, call back and talk to a different representative as well as escalate to a supervisor. Keep escalating until you get a yes and find that person who will advocate for you.

Most of the time you will succeed, depending on the insurance plan and insurance company. Even if you fail and don't manage to get the insurance company to pay for some or all of the entire pump, you will have succeeded as a parent.

Just as you need the support of your child's doctor in this process, it is important to support your child even if you think they will fail because once they leave home, they will have to become their own advocate. It is important to be an example for them by supporting them and advocating for them.

In Tom's case, he is one of a handful of teenagers who openly wanted to improve their management. Most teens want to have good management but don't know how to go about it. Even if it seems impossible, support them and fight for and advocate for your child. They will take that life lesson into the world. You will feel more assured that your child will manage their diabetes without your supervision.

CLINICAL ADVICE

There are benefits of using an insulin pump. The options available with different pumps and the importance of working with your healthcare team are discussed below.

Pumps will increase your child's ability to make more informed choices around how much or how little insulin to bolus. They help improve blood sugar stability. Pumps will also decrease your child's HbA1c results. Every bit helps.

The data entered into the pump and collected by the pump tells you when insulin is still on board, allowing people on the pump to make more informed decisions about how much insulin to give (or not).

When you have both a continuous glucose monitor (CGM) and an insulin pump, management becomes increasingly easier as your child and you become more skilled at using the CGM and the pump. They are highly recommended to use together.

You need to know your options when picking your child's pump. Not all pumps come in different colors, like with the CGMs. When buying an insulin pump, it is important to look at all available options.

Depending on your experience with pumps, you may choose a different pump from what your child's endocrinologist or certified diabetes educator recommends. The decision needs to meet your child's individual needs for your child's unique circumstance.

If your child regularly breaks their phone, then how durable the pump is will be a major factor. When your child's average daily insulin usage is 100 units of insulin, it doesn't make sense to choose a pump that only holds up to 180 or 200 units when there are pumps that can hold 480 units of insulin. It is important to think about whether this option makes sense for your child's needs and lifestyle. If your child is on the swim team, à waterproof insulin pump might be required.

The Closed Loop

Hopefully, by the time you read this, more than one company will offer a pump with a closed loop system, with more options and better accuracy. A closed-loop pump has a built-in continuous glucose meter that tells the pump what your blood sugar is, allowing the device to make corrective boluses or reduce basil delivery for you. The closed-loop system helps stabilize blood sugar throughout the day while preventing high and low blood sugars during the night.

With these systems, you need to consider the accuracy of the CGM the pump uses, as well as the target basal rate. Presently the only closed-loop system on the market is designed to keep the basal rate at 120 mg/dL, and for someone whose blood sugars are well managed, this basal rate might be too high. Please consult your endocrinologist or certified diabetes educator to discuss the benefits and drawbacks of this system for your child.

At present, the closed-loop system has the benefit of providing corrective boluses during the night to keep blood sugar levels on target.

Some Unique Pump Options

Some pumps use a monitor remote that controls nearly all pump functions: delivering a bolus, monitoring pump stats, and confirming alarms as well as warnings. Other pumps have a built-in CGM that uses a sensor to wirelessly transmit glucose readings throughout the day. This setup allows the consumer with diabetes to carry one less device. Some pumps use icons instead of words in the display as well as a pump without tubing.

Table 11.1. Pump Option

Closed Loop	How accurate is the continuous glucose meter?
Size and Weight	Ranges from 2.29 oz to 4.4 oz with battery and full reservoir.
Reservoir Size	How much insulin does the pump hold? Pump cartridge sizes range from 180 to 480 units.
Color	What colors does the pump come in?
Screen	How big is the screen? Can I clearly read it? Is it backlit so I can read in the dark? Monochrome or color?
Display	Is it a touch screen display?
Infusion Set	Is the cannula insertion device manual or automatic?
Angle of Insertion	Discuss with your endocrinologist as to what angle will work best with your child's body type.
Basal Range	Some pumps go from 0.01 to 25 units per hour in 0.01-unit increments. Where other pumps have less flexibility, 0.5 to 10 units per hour in 0.1-unit increments.
Bolus Range	Some pumps deliver as little as 0.025 to a maximum of 60 units delivered in unit increments (speed of insulin delivery) with a minimum of 0.01 to as fast as 1-unit increments. Does the pump allow for insulin-to-carb ratios in fractions of grams or insulin-to-carb ratios in whole units only?
Record Events	Do you have the ability to manually enter insulin, exercise, carbs, or other health data?
Alarms	How adjustable are they? Can you set the alarms for different times throughout the day and night, different sounds for each alarm, and how loud the alarms are?
Waterproof	Is the pump waterproof, and do you need it to be?
Batteries	What type of battery is required, and is it rechargeable? How long does the charge last?
Data Collection	Do you need to own a computer, or is there an app on your phone that will upload the pump data?
Upgrade	Is there a program in place that allows you to upgrade when a newer model comes on the market?
Customer Service	Does the company that makes the pump have a good track record responding to requests and questions?

Make sure to go online and look up the most recent consumer guide, since technology changes very rapidly and more options might be available by the time you read this.

Medical Consultation

As with the CGM, it is important to consult with your endocrinologist or certified diabetes educator when choosing what pump to purchase. There are required procedures in place that have to be followed. Some health insurance companies might require three months of documented blood sugar results along with a prescription from your endocrinologist plus additional paperwork.

Have your healthcare team help you decide on what is the most appropriate pump for your child's needs. Check to see whether your healthcare providers or medical suppliers can contact your insurance on your behalf to obtain the necessary documentation and check which pumps are covered. If they won't contact your insurance, it is important that you contact your health insurance company, as some health insurances cover only approved pumps.

The process of getting your child's pump, as previously mentioned, may go smoothly, or you may have to advocate. If your doctor prescribes a pump, it means that the device is medically necessary. However, some insurance companies will approve only certain pump brands, but they can't deny it altogether.

They may try to deny based on the blood sugar results from the collected blood glucose diary you provided the insurance company. In that case, your doctor might have to go to bat for you and contact your insurance company.

Regardless of whether everything goes smoothly, it is worth fighting for, so don't give up. Insurance companies like saying no, but you can escalate all the way to the CEO. I wish you the best of luck.

Epilogue

I want to share a little of my story. I did a lot of crazy, silly, and (some might say) stupid things while growing up with diabetes. I believe all children do, not intentionally but because we learn as we grow. During my childhood, I experienced three hypoglycemic episodes that resulted in trips to the hospital and unstable blood sugars from diagnosis through college (detailed in chapter 7).

I liked binging on candy, and high blood sugars were the norm during my childhood. The high blood sugar caused depression, increased levels of anxiety, emotional instability, lots of dehydration, and many other physical and emotional issues. I was angry that I had diabetes, that I was different from my friends, and I felt very alone living with the illness.

Due to poor diabetes control, I was always reacting to my environment instead of being able to think things through. I ended up pushing all the people who could help me away. I figured I was in control of diabetes when in reality I was far from it.

At twelve, I started going to therapy to deal with the drama in my life (everyone has some amount), but I never talked about diabetes. Just resolving the issues I was having with my family and the emotions I was going through helped me make room in my head for diabetes self-management.

It was still difficult. I am not even going to get into the management challenges that college life brought me. It would have been nice to have someone to talk to about those challenges, but there was no therapist specializing in diabetes back then, unlike now.

I fully believe that therapy is a great source of support, and I found relief from the mini traumas that come with diabetes, including daily frustration. I know! It surprised me as well. I thought I was insane, but I wasn't. Most people who go to therapy are not crazy. They just need nonbiased support to deal with the issues they are going through or live with every day, like chronic illness or family stress.

Getting help takes a lot of strength because many people are taught and encouraged to be independent, even if we need the support of others. Difficulty getting help is especially true for those dealing with a chronic condition like diabetes. Admitting that we can't do it alone anymore takes a lot of courage and strength.

For my journey in psychotherapy, since I had been on my own for my whole life, I had difficulty admitting that I couldn't do it alone, but therapy helped me realize it can be easier. With support from a nonbiased individual, like a therapist, it gets easier—not instantly, but it does.

Some therapists did not work for my needs or personality. Eventually, I found a good therapist who created a safe, nonbiased environment where I could talk about my issues without having to worry about policing or judgment from my family or friends. I developed Diabetes-Focused Psychotherapy as a place where you can get diabetes management and emotional support without having to deal with being judged or getting into an argument.

While creating Diabetes-Focused Psychotherapy, I found many techniques to manage diabetes or the emotions that come from it. Many management methods were unknown to me, and I found that to be true for other people living with diabetes diagnosed decades ago. Before studying to become a certified diabetes educator or developing Diabetes-Focused Psychotherapy, I thought I knew everything about diabetes.

After years of helping people living with diabetes, I look back and realize how little I knew back then. There is always more to learn and no limit to how much we can grow, whether it is diabetes management or living a happier, well-balanced life.

We are always learning new things every day, and psychotherapy helps people gain new levels of clarity about their relationships and themselves so they can learn how to manage life with less negative emotions and frustration.

Growing up, I never wanted to talk about my diabetes. I would say to myself, "No one will understand what it is like living with diabetes!" I was wrong. Eventually, I found a therapist who was empathetic to what I was going through, and it only took two decades to share my diabetes-specific feelings.

After so long, a big weight was lifted off my shoulders, and management started getting easier. Psychotherapy helped me. In turn, I decided to help others living with diabetes, and that is how I ended up talking about diabetes and developing Diabetes-Focused Psychotherapy.

Unlike the insensitive discussions around my diabetes growing up, these conversations are constructive and helpful to my clients. I have also learned so much from my clients: tips, tricks, and unique ways to manage. In return, I now have a wealth of knowledge beyond my formal education that I can pass along to my incoming clients.

After all these years, why do I keep going back for my therapy? It's no longer about feeling anxious, frustrated, angry, and depressed or the myriad of other issues I was going through as a child or young adult. I found therapy to be a great support: reducing stress, providing clarity, and helping to keep diabetes burnout at bay.

So, I went from a death sentence to a happier life with a personally satisfying career helping others living with diabetes. Thanks to my mom, because she decided to send me to therapy. I didn't want to go, but I am grateful I did. Go figure.

I have watched many parents of children with diabetes in my private practice struggle but never give up. The fight to raise a child is demanding.

Raising a child with diabetes is filled with a lot more work that is physically, emotionally, and mentally demanding. The job of the parent who has a child with diabetes is never-ending. It never stops or turns off.

In addition to dealing with your needs and feelings as individuals, you the parent have to remain stable so your child can grow up healthy and strong. The tremendous job of raising a child with diabetes is twenty-four hours a day, seven days a week. That is why, if you or your child are struggling, it is important to get help.

I want to thank all of you for reading my book and sharing in my clients' and my experiences growing up. I hope you took a lot away to help you on your journey as a parent of a child living with diabetes.

For more on Diabetes-Focused Psychotherapy and how it might help you and your family, go to my website: www.diabetictalks.com.

Appendix A

100 Dos and Don'ts to Make Your Child Smile!

DOS

1. Give them a hug and kiss.
2. Spend time with them.
3. Give them the ability to choose (within reason).
4. Buy a toy for your child because they are managing their diabetes *better* (not perfectly).
5. Compliment them when their blood glucose is good.
6. When blood sugars are not so good, remind them that it is okay because it is normal.
7. Encourage self-thought.
8. Tell them that they are good enough once a week.
9. Remind them often that they are not alone.
10. When they make a mistake, stay calm.
11. Remind them that making mistakes are part of being human.
12. Praise or reward them when they correct the mistake.
13. Tell them that having diabetes is not their fault; it just happens.
14. Support their feelings by saying, "I feel that way at times too."
15. Encourage them to share their feelings.
16. Allow them to be part of the decision making around diabetes management.
17. Encourage them to share good and bad feelings.

18. Validate their feelings by saying, "I can understand why you feel that way."
19. Plan for alone time with your child weekly and stick to it.
20. Let them choose the family activity once in a while.
21. Allow them to go out on a school night with a friend when they are managing their blood glucose well.
22. Give positive praise for controlling how they react to emotional ups and downs (such as "way to check your blood sugar when you are feeling bad").
23. Every now and then, give a treat for behaving appropriately.
24. Take care of their diabetes management together.
25. Talk about other things besides their diabetes.
26. Be flexible when plans change due to their diabetes.
27. Tell them it is okay to say things like "I forgot my shot [or my diabetic supplies]" or "Can we stop? I need to test or go to the bathroom for the tenth time in an hour."
28. Give them alone time (people are always focusing on them because of their diabetes).
29. Share how you feel (within reason and age appropriateness).
30. Teach them how to play a sport.
31. Play with them (yes, that means your kid might beat you at a Nintendo game).
32. Say yes to the ice cream man once in a while.
33. Ask them if they would like to play a game out of the blue.
34. Use their advice (when appropriate).
35. Keep reminding yourself that they are not mini adults.
36. Allow them to run and play (where appropriate).
37. Tell them good things you remember from your childhood.
38. Put down your phone and be present and attentive.
39. Climb a tree with them.
40. Skip stones with them.
41. Share your hobbies.
42. Let them share their hobbies with you.

43. Do their chores with them once in a while.
44. Show love through your behaviors.
45. Help them with homework (do not do their homework for them).
46. Put the work away and be in the present with them.
47. Read to your child.
48. Have a movie popcorn night.
49. Quit smoking.
50. Learn something new together.
51. Get them the pet they keep asking for.
52. Let them pick out their own clothes.
53. Inform them of decisions that impact them before you do it and ask their opinion.
54. Respect their opinions and views.
55. Explain what you are doing and why.
56. Include them in family decisions.
57. Compromise.
58. Be the parent, not a friend.
59. Tickle their feet.
60. Raspberry their stomach.
61. Use the adaptive style of diabetes management.
62. Work on reducing your frustration levels around your child's management.
63. Work on reducing your guilt around their diabetes.
64. Accept where your child is, as far as telling others about their diabetes (within reason; you are still going to have to tell adults who interact with your child).
65. Do chores together like raking leaves.
66. Rake some leaves into a giant pile and both of you jump in (counterproductive, yes, but fun as hell—hell yes).
67. Explain why you are making decisions that involve them.
68. You do as you say you are going to do.
69. Help them manage their feelings around having diabetes.

70. Take care of the pet together (you both might walk the dog together and talk).
71. Take the time to listen to them.
72. Accept their personality (they are not mini versions of you).
73. Positive reinforcement (tell them they are doing good).
74. Involve the whole family in therapy to discuss issues that cause fights between your child with diabetes and the rest of the family.
75. Get them therapy help so they come to accept their diabetes.

DON'TS
1. Make a big deal about their diabetes.
2. Punish your child for high blood sugars.
3. Disregard their feelings.
4. Yell at them for being a kid.
5. Show anger or frustration over changing plans due to your child's diabetes.
6. Blame your child's diabetes.
7. Smoke cigarettes or use other nicotine products.
8. Abuse alcohol.
9. Use illicit drugs.
10. Constantly talk about their diabetes.
11. Ignore feelings around having diabetes.
12. Fight (talk things out instead).
13. Become obsessed with their diabetes.
14. Rebuff the fact that they have diabetes.
15. Be overly strict when managing your child's diabetes.
16. Relinquish management of your child's diabetes (even older children need some support).
17. Ignore the fact that your child has diabetes.
18. Show frustration in general.
19. Use a methodical style of diabetes management.
20. Use an inadequate style of diabetes management.
21. Choose work over your child.

22. Isolate your child from their peers.
23. Worry about fluctuating blood sugars (it's normal).
24. Drive them to school when they say, "It's embarrassing!"
25. Talk about their diabetes in front of their friends.

Appendix B

Resources

MENTAL HEALTH

ADA Mental Health Directory is a place to find a diabetes-friendly psychotherapist in your neighborhood. https://professional.diabetes.org/ada-mental-health-provider-directory

The *DiabeticMinds* blog was created by psychotherapist Eliot LeBow, LCSW, CDE, who is a certified diabetes educator diagnosed with type 1 diabetes at age six. The author discusses a wide range of topics from mental health to diabetes management in easy-to-understand terminology. www.diabeticminds.com

DiabeticTalks is Eliot LeBow's website, helping people with diabetes thrive. It has many resources to help adults, children, and families master the emotional, cognitive, and management challenges of diabetes. https://www.diabetictalks.com

ARTICLES

"Demystifying Psychotherapy: Helping You Navigate the Process of Getting Emotional Help!" is an article on the website DiabeticTalks to help people understand the process of looking for a good mental health professional. https://www.diabetictalks.com/assets/demystifying_therapy.pdf

"Depression Overview, Diagnosis & Treatment" is a section on the website DiabeticTalks that provides much-needed information about the impact of depression on diabetes and the treatment needed to reduce its effects. https://www.diabetictalks.com/depression-overview.html

"Resolve ADHD to Improve Diabetes Self-Management" (May 2016) is an article in *Endocrine Today* about the impact of attention deficit/hyperactivity disorder (ADHD) on diabetes self-management and how to reduce the effects of ADHD. http://dld.bz/gN2Hz

"Unraveling the Diabetic Binge: Solving the Uncontrollable Urge to Eat and Eat Despite the Consequences" is an article on DiabeticTalks that looks at the physical reasons why people with diabetes binge eat when hypoglycemic. https://www.diabetictalks.com/assets/unravelingthediabetic-binge.pdf

Other mental health articles: https://www.diabetictalks.com/articles.html

NEWLY DIAGNOSED
Diabetes Research Institute offers emotional support and practical tips from professionals and fellow parents who live with diabetes day to day. https://www.diabetesresearch.org/PEP-Squad

JDRF Bag of Hope includes Rufus the Bear with Diabetes and many other things to help children recently diagnosed. https://www.jdrf.org/t1d-resources/newly-diagnosed/children/bag-of-hope

Friends for Life is an annual conference held in Orlando each July for parents, teens, siblings, and more. Other programs are offered throughout the year as well, such as technology programs and overseas programs. www.childrenwithdiabetes.com/activities/

Understanding Diabetes, 13th ed. by Peter H. Chase is an instruction manual for families on the management of diabetes.

Bright Spots and Landmines: The Diabetes Guide I Wish Someone Had Handed Me by Adam Brown is an actionable guide around food choice, mindset, exercise, and sleep strategies that have positively impacted his diabetes—and hopefully yours too!

DIABETES AT SCHOOL
This guide includes an extensive amount of information on diabetes management while at school. A must-read guide to help your child and their teachers interact and react accordingly to your and your child's needs while at school. https://www.diabetictalks.com/ndep-school-guide.html

Children with Diabetes provides examples of various versions of the 504 plans based on grade level at school. http://www.childrenwithdiabetes.com/504

Living with T1 Diabetes: JDRF School Section includes its School Advisory Kit and information about your child's rights. https://www.jdrf.org/t1d-resources/living-with-t1d/school

The American Diabetes Association Written Care Plans: http://www.diabetes.org/living-with-diabetes/parents-and-kids/diabetes-care-at-school/written-care-plans

CAMP

ADA Camps provides a unique community-based experience for kids and their families, where they can grow together. http://www.diabetes.org/in-my-community/diabetes-camp

Diabetes Education and Camping Association provides a search engine to help parents find diabetes-friendly camps. https://www.diabetes-camps.org

Riding on Insulin are design camps that are held around the world annually for kids with diabetes who want to snowboard or ski. Run by world-class snowboarder and person with T1D Sean Busby. www.ridingoninsulin.org

The Barton Center for Diabetes/Camp Joslin improves the lives of children with insulin-dependent diabetes through education, recreation, and support programs that inspire and empower. http://www.barton-center.org

BLOGS

Parenting Children with Diabetes was created by Eliot LeBow, LCSW, CDE, as a continuation of the book *Parenting Children with Diabetes.* www.raisingdiabetes.com

Arden's Day is a type 1 parenting blog written by the author of *Life Is Short, Laundry Is Eternal,* a stay-at-home father raising a daughter who was diagnosed with type 1 diabetes at the age of two. www.ardensday.com

Ask Manny Hernandez is a blog written by Manny Hernandez, a social media expert, leading diabetes advocate, and founder/past president of the Diabetes Hands Foundation. He writes about his experiences with diabetes and diabetes management and posts pictures. http://askmanny.com/

A Sweet Life is a blog that provides lots of tools and advice to thrive with diabetes. Aside from its personal story, the blog offers recipes, travel tips, personal stories from guest bloggers, updates on research, and more. https://asweetlife.org/

Bitter-Sweet was created because life with diabetes isn't all bad. The author is a caring individual and a knitter who lives with type 1 diabetes. She is not a medical professional, nor does she give medical advice; she states, "I'm just a girl sharing my thoughts and experiences with diabetes." www.bittersweetdiabetes.com

D-Mom is the online shorthand for the mother of a child who has diabetes. Read about the author's family as their story unfolds. www.d-mom. com

DiabeticMinds was created by a psychotherapist who is a certified diabetes educator diagnosed with type 1 diabetes at age six. The author discusses a wide range of topics from mental health to diabetes management in easy-to-understand terminology. www.diabeticminds.com

Diabetes DAD was created by a father of two children living with type 1 diabetes who is an advocate in the world of diabetes to help educate and inspire all those who are parents or who live with diabetes. www. diabetesdad.org

DiabetesMine is written by a group of bloggers and provides innovation, information, advocacy, and tips on living with type 1 diabetes. www. diabetesmine.com

Diabetesaliciousness is written by an adult with type 1 diabetes who spreads diabetes validation through humor, ownership, and advocacy. The writer is busting diabetes myths and perpetuating diabetes realities. http://diabetesaliciousness.blogspot.com

dLife is written by a group of bloggers to educate, empower, and encourage you to take control of your diabetes. https://dlife.com/diabetesblog/

Our Diabetic Life imparts wisdom and insight from a mom raising three boys with type 1 diabetes. www.ourdiabeticlife.com

Scott's Diabetes: Helping You See Your Strengths brings an honest and open account of his life with diabetes while providing insight and accurate input on eating issues, struggles, and successes. www.scottsdiabetes.com

Six Until Me was developed by an adult with type 1 diabetes who discusses daily living with diabetes in a down-to-earth way. www.sixuntilme.com

Sweetly Voiced is the personal blog of Melissa Lee, the current director of Community Relations at Bigfoot BioMedical. A self-described "diabetic, a singer, and a mommy," Melissa Lee shares her experiences with diabetes technology, advocacy work, HbA1c history, and more. http://www.sweetlyvoiced.com

Texting My Pancreas supplies the reader with advice and insight from a woman who has grown up with type 1 diabetes. www.textingmypancreas.com

PHONE APPLICATIONS

Diabetes:M delivers one-click diabetes management by calculating regular and prolonged insulin boluses while offering an extensive nutrition database. The app can set blood sugar reminders and log exercise time. It also works with different glucometers and insulin pumps to analyze values from imported data.

Glooko allows the user to view their progress through charts and keep track of their history while monitoring medications, carb intake, and more. It integrates data from most continuous glucose monitors, blood glucose meters, insulin pumps, and fitness trackers.

Health2Sync has the unique feature of helping you create a diabetes support community with your friends or family as well as practical functions like documenting your sugar readings, weight, and other factors that affect diabetes. This app also syncs with Bluetooth health devices.

mySugr aims to make diabetes less difficult by syncing with other devices to help you monitor weight, basal rates, and sugar levels. mySugr helps users log in their data through notifications that appear on their phone—assisting users to stay on top of their diabetes and giving users the ability to report critical facts to their doctors.

WEBSITES/ORGANIZATIONS
American Association of Diabetes Educators is a multidisciplinary association of healthcare professionals dedicated to integrating self-management as a critical outcome in the care of people with diabetes and related conditions. www.diabeteseducator.org

American Diabetes Association (ADA) is a national nonprofit health organization providing diabetes research, information, and advocacy. www.diabetes.org

Beyond Type 1 is educating the global community about diabetes, as well as providing resources and supporting those living with type 1 diabetes. Beyond Type 1 is bridging the gap from diagnosis to cure, empowering people to live well today and funding a better tomorrow. www.beyondtype1.org

Children with Diabetes is a leading destination on the internet for families dealing with type 1 diabetes and perhaps the largest and most respected online diabetes community. Parents and teens alike can find information, guidance, and real-time support. www.childrenwithdiabetes.com

Diabetes Daily is an online community for people living with diabetes. They believe that everyone with diabetes can live healthy, happy, and hopeful lives. Every day, they help connect people with diabetes, empower them to manage their condition successfully, and advocate for their interests. Their most popular tools include online educational programs, one of the largest diabetes forums, and an extensive collection of original recipes. www.diabetesdaily.com

diaTribe is an online community and website geared toward all people who are living with diabetes. They provide education, awareness, advocacy, and advice as well as information about the latest diabetes workshops and conferences. https://diatribe.org/

Insulin Nation is a news platform for people with type 1 diabetes. The site curates the latest research, technology, treatments, policy, and advocacy updates all in one place. http://www.insulinnation.com/

Joslin Diabetes Center is an affiliate of Harvard Medical School as well as a one-of-a-kind institution on the front lines of the world epidemic of diabetes—leading the battle to conquer diabetes in all of its forms through cutting-edge research and innovative approaches to clinical care and education. www.joslin.org

Juvenile Diabetes Research Foundation (JDRF) is the leading global organization focused on type 1 diabetes research. www.jdrf.org

tuDiabetes is a space on the web where people with diabetes or their loved ones can find support, help each other, and share their experiences and what they do every day to stay healthy with this condition. www.tudiabetes.org

TypeOneNation is JDRF's vibrant social network for people with type 1 diabetes (T1D), their families, and friends. Members of this diverse and lively community exchange information, answers, and support. www.typeonenation.org

TWEETERS

DiabeticTalks is tweeted out by Eliot LeBow, LCSW, CDE, who is a diabetes-focused psychotherapist and certified diabetes educator as well as a type 1 diabetic since 1977. He uses his online platform to help people living with diabetes thrive through providing information and guidance on how to manage the emotional issues like diabetes distress, other mental health issues, and the daily trauma of living with diabetes. Follow him @DiabeticTalks

Arden's Day T1D posted by Scott Brenner helps parents facing the unique challenges of raising kids with type 1 diabetes. He began blogging about his experience as a dad of a type 1 child in 2007. Follow him @ardensday

Beyond Type 1 is an online community that shares inspirational memes, links to the latest articles, and more. You can use it to find others with type 1 diabetes or to find daily motivation and support. Follow them @BeyondType1

Children with Diabetes shares news about important advocacy work while retweeting some great information to help families with type 1 diabetes stay connected. Tweet them @cwdiabetes

Diabetes Daily offers the latest in diabetes news along with practical advice on diet and exercise. Follow them @diabetesdaily

Diabetes Health is an excellent resource for daily news, podcasts, and personal stories about living with diabetes. Follow them @DiabetesHealth

Diabetes Research Institute provides the latest developments in the world of diabetes research. Their feed has news about their most recent efforts as well as information on what is going on with scientists and researchers. Follow them @Diabetes_DRI

Diabetes Self-Management helps people with diabetes management and all that goes with it. Their feed is a great place to find the latest articles on recipes and dietary advice to medical emergency preparedness. Follow them @ManageDiabetes

Diabetes UK is the leading diabetes organization in the UK, sharing news, research, and advocacy work as well as retweeting followers' personal photographs and stories. Follow them @DiabetesUK

DiabetesMine is managed by three contributors, Amy Tenderich, Mike Hoskins, and Rachel Kestetter. It's an excellent resource for advice and the latest news. Follow them @DiabetesMine

diaTribe is an online community and website geared toward all people who are living with diabetes. They provide education, awareness, advocacy, and advice as well as information about the latest diabetes workshops and conferences. Follow them @diaTribeNews

The International Diabetes Federation works to foster government support for diabetes research worldwide. Its Twitter account shares information on the impact of diabetes, including infographics and links to their articles. Follow them @IntDiabetesFed

JDRF is a long-standing organization that advocates for diabetes awareness and research, with a focus on type 1 diabetes. It hosts Twitter chats about diabetes research and shares the latest news in diabetes, while providing unique and helpful information for families living with diabetes. Follow them @JDRF

Six Until Me is written by Kerri Morrone Sparling, who was diagnosed at six years old and now writes a blog also called *Six Until Me*. On Twitter, Kerri shares links to her latest blog posts, plus news stories and tips. Follow her @sixuntilme

tuDiabetes is a nonprofit that works to connect and inspire people living with diabetes. Its Twitter account provides personal stories and educational links. Follow them @diabeteshf

BOOKS

Coco and Goofy's Goofy Day by Susan Amerikaner is a fun, free online book to help children manage peer issues in an imaginative way. The book is published by Disney Press, which provides many excellent, fun, free online books with audio recordings to help children manage the challenges of diabetes. https://www.t1everydaymagic.com/books/

Diabetes Burnout: What to Do When You Can't Take It Anymore by William Polonsky, PhD, is a little dated but remains a go-to source for information on dealing with diabetes burnout.

Life Is Short, Laundry Is Eternal is by Scott Benner, who with his colloquial wisdom will warm your heart while challenging your ideas about parenting and gender roles in today's households. Scott discusses being a stay-at-home dad and balancing family life and his daughter Arden's diabetes, creating an honest portrait of the modern family.

Pumping Insulin: Everything You Need for Success with an Insulin Pump by John Walsh has been referred to as the "bible of pumping" by many and is an excellent resource for people using insulin pumps.

Think Like a Pancreas: A Practical Guide to Managing Diabetes with Insulin by Gary Scheiner provides tips and details on managing insulin in the real world.

Transitions in Care: Meeting the Challenges of Type 1 Diabetes in Young Adults by Howard Wolpert, MD; Barbara Anderson, PhD; and Jill Weissberg-Benchell, PhD, serves as a coaching manual for healthcare providers and parents. The book is a guide to self-care and independence for young adults with diabetes.

The Everything Parent's Guide to Children with Juvenile Diabetes by Moira McCarthy covers the basics of diabetes and helps lay a foundation for proper management.

The Ultimate Guide to Accurate Carb Counting by Gary Scheiner tells you everything you need to accurately keep track of your carb intake, including the underlying rationale for and the theory behind carb counting, as well as explanations of simple to advanced techniques.

Appendix C

504 Sample

For a more comprehensive form, visit https://www.diabetictalks.com/ndep-school-guide.html

Fill out prior to parent conference:

Date: _____ Valid for the Current School/ Year: _____/_____

Child's Name _____ Date of Birth _____

Mother's Name _____ Father's Name _____

Contact: please include name, phone numbers, relationship, location, legal authority to act in an emergency (list by call order):

1.
2.
3.
4.
5.

Primary Care Physician:

Name: _____ Phone: _____

Other Health Providers:

Name: _____ Specialty: _____ Phone: _____

Name: _____ Specialty: _____ Phone: _____

Name: _____ Specialty: _____ Phone: _____

Monitoring

Usual blood glucose monitoring times:
Before: ☐ Breakfast ☐ Lunch ☐ PE ☐ Dismissal **After:** ☐ Breakfast ☐ Lunch
  ☐ PE ☐ As needed for low or high blood glucose
  ☐ Other: _____

Where should your child monitor their blood glucose (classroom, health office, etc.)?

Blood Glucose Goals: Between _____ and _____.
Lows:
If below _____, please do the following:

If below _____, please do the following:

Call parent if below _____
Signs/symptoms of your child's low blood glucose: _____

Highs:
If above_____, please do the following:

If above_____, please do the following:

Measure ketones when your child's blood glucose gets to _____
Call parent if blood glucose gets above _____
Signs/symptoms of your child's high blood glucose:

Insulin

Will daily insulin injections be needed in school? YES / NO
Will insulin injections be needed in school at any other time? YES / NO
Does your child use a pump? YES / NO
If YES to any of the above, please elaborate; identify time, amount, and circumstances
  for administering insulin.

Other information you feel is necessary to assist school staff around insulin
  maintenance.

Food:
Will the child participate in school breakfast and/or school lunch? YES / NO
If yes, will modifications to the regular menu be needed? YES / NO
What are their usual times for meals/snacks?
_____ Breakfast _____ Mid-morning _____ Lunch _____ Mid-afternoon
_____ Supper _____ Bedtime

Exercise

What are your child's favorite physical activities?

_____

_____

Will your child participate in school sports? YES / NO
Your child's role in diabetes self-management: (check all that apply)

▫ Does it alone	▫ Adjusts food based on result
▫ Does it with supervision	▫ Adjusts insulin based on result
▫ Helps parent	▫ Knows which foods to limit
▫ Parent does it	▫ Can adjust the amount of food
▫ Pricks finger	▫ Selects insulin injection site
▫ Puts strip in monitor	▫ Prepares for injection, selects
▫ Reads monitor	site
▫ Records result	▫ Sets bolus (premeal)
▫ Helps plan meals	▫ Sets bolus (lower high BG)
▫ Injects insulin	▫ Sets temporary basal rate
▫ Measures insulin	▫ Determines amount of insulin
▫ Adjusts pump settings	▫ Measures ketones

Other:

_____

_____

_____

Parties and food-related events

Should we contact you before each event? YES / NO
Additional instructions:

_____

_____

_____

Emergencies:
What constitutes an emergency for your child?

_____

_____

_____

What should the school's role be in an emergency?
Other requests:

_____

_____

_____

OTHER SECTION 504 PLAN RESOURCES

National Institute of Diabetes and Digestive and Kidney Diseases (NI-DDK): https://www.diabetictalks.com/ndep-school-guide.html

The American Diabetes Association Written Care Plans: http://www.diabetes.org/living-with-diabetes/parents-and-kids/diabetes-care-at-school/written-care-plans

Bibliography

American Association of Diabetes Educators. Updated January 2019. https://www.diabeteseducator.org.

American Diabetes Association. Updated January 2019. http://www.diabetes.org.

Brandell, Jerrold. *Theory & Practice in Clinical Social Work*. 2nd edition. New York: Free Press, 2010.

Broderick, Pamela, and Christina Weston. "Family Therapy with a Depressed Adolescent." *Psychiatry (Edgmont)* 6, no. 1 (January 2009): 32–37.

Corey, Gerald. *Theory and Practice of Counseling and Psychotherapy*. 8th edition. California: Brooks/Cole, 2008.

Cornell, Susan, et al. *The Art and Science of Diabetes Self-Management Education Desk Reference*. 4th edition. Chicago: America Association of Diabetes Educators, 2017.

Joslin Diabetes Center. Updated January 2019. http://www.joslin.org.

Juvenile Diabetes Research Foundation (2018). Updated January 2019. https://www.jdrf.org.

Katon, Wayne, et al. "Association of Depression with Increased Risk of Severe Hypoglycemic Episodes in Patients with Diabetes." *Annals of Family*

Medicine 11, no. 3 (May/June 2013): 245–50. https://doi.org/10.1370/afm.1501.

McCrimmon, Rory, et al. "Diabetes and Cognitive Dysfunction." *Lancet* 379, no. 9833 (June 2012): 2291–99. https://doi.org/10.1016/S0140-6736(12)60360-2.

Miller, Williams, and Stephen Rollnick. *Motivational Interviewing: Preparing People for Change.* New York: Guilford Press, 2012.

Nichols, Michael, and Sean Davis. *Family Therapy Concepts and Methods.* 11th edition. Boston: Pearson, 2017.

Northam, Elisabeth, et al. "Neuropsychological Profiles of Children with Type 1 Diabetes 6 Years after Disease Onset." *Diabetes Care* 24, no. 9 (September 2001): 1541–46. https://doi.org/10.2337/diacare.24.9.1541.

Perantie, Dana, et al. "Prospectively Determined Impact of Type 1 Diabetes on Brain Volume During Development." *Diabetes* 60, no. 11 (November 2011): 3006–14. https://doi.org/10.2337/db11-0589.

Polonsky, William. *Diabetes Burnout: What to Do When You Can't Take It Anymore.* Alexandria, VA: American Diabetes Association, 1999.

Steinberg, Marc, and William Miller. *Motivational Interviewing for People with Diabetes.* New York: Guilford Press, 2015.

Index